Many of the designations used by manufacturers and sellers to distinguish their products are claimed by trademarks. Where those designations appear in this book and the authors were aware of a trademark claim, the designations have been printed in initial caps (e.g., Proventil).

A C K N O W L E D G E M E N T S

We would like to acknowledge and thank Pam Schmidt, our Art Director, whose vision, creativity, and organization made this project possible. Special thanks to Felix Frazier and Becky Bertino, who believed in our concept and in us. Many thanks to Daphne Terrell, Elsie Brenner, and Linda Smith for their critical eyes and gentle reviews.

ISBN 0-9718120-9-8
ISBN 0-9718120-2-0 (Child/Parent Health Set)

LCCN: 2002102112
Library of Congress Cataloging-in-Publication Data is available.

10 9 8 7 6 5 4 3 2 1
Printed in the United States of America

Cover and Book Design by:
   Thumbnails
   208 Ware Drive
   Buda, TX 78610

Printed by Clarke Printing Company

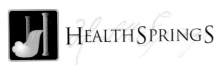

Published by:
   HealthSprings, LLC
   1759 Grandstand
   San Antonio, TX 78238

Zoey and the Zones™, Zoey™ and Light Buddy™ are registered trademarks of Zoey, L.P.

"As a practicing pediatric physician and children's hospital administrator, I am well aware of the magnitude of problems caused by childhood asthma. This workbook on asthma is long overdue and has the potential to help families and children who will be fortunate enough to have access to it. It is accurate, entertaining, educational, and easy to understand. All of these characteristics should make it a staple for years to come."

Richard S. Wayne, M.D., Vice President and CEO
Christus Santa Rosa Children's Hospital

"Zoey and the Zones takes critical asthma information and translates it into a fun learning experience for kids. The message of this book is powerful yet is delivered in a manner that children understand and will find entertaining. This beloved character provides children with the tools they need to cope with this chronic and challenging illness."

David Dukes, Chairman
CHOC Foundation for Children

"As an educator of respiratory therapists, I believe this workbook can serve as an excellent tool for use by therapists, nurses, pharmacists, and physicians involved in the care of children with asthma. The text is superb and the graphics are engaging. A wonderful book for young children and their parents, who are looking for tools that will help them manage this chronic disease."

David C. Shelledy, PhD, RRT
Chair, Department of Respiratory Care
The University of Texas Health Science Center at San Antonio

"As a practicing pharmacist for over twenty years and as a policymaker, I am excited about the easy, enjoyable format of Zoey and the Zones. Families and patients with asthma will benefit greatly from this teaching tool."

Leticia Van De Putte, RPh
Texas State Senator

"As a mother with three young children, life can be very busy. Add to that a chronic lung disease, times three, and you can easily feel overwhelmed. I enjoyed reading Zoey and the Zones with my children. It was a fun read written with a wide age range of children in mind. Zoey and the Zones is also a guide to assist in making management plans for your specific individual needs. This comprehensive book is wonderful for the person (or caregiver) just diagnosed with asthma, as well as a tool for people currently controlling their symptoms. Asthma is manageable. Learn as much as you can and follow your plan. Enjoy your life to the fullest!"

Jo Anne Naro, Mother of Three Children with Asthma
Medfield, Massachusetts

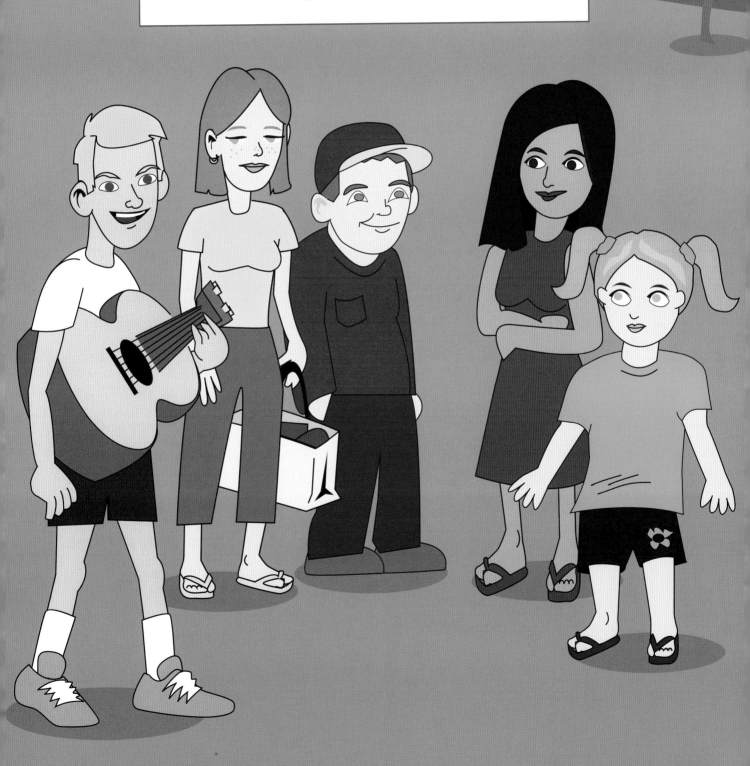

FOREWORD

Today, with asthma on the rise, there are many books available on the subject. Most are written by clinicians for clinicians. We felt there was a need for a comprehensive workbook that addresses all of the elements encountered by a child with asthma and his family.

Zoey and the Zones is an interactive workbook with sections specifically designed for the parent, followed by related activities for children. The book needs to be studied and completed as a family activity. We recommend that you take your time studying and understanding all of the information provided in each section. A good schedule for you and your child would be to complete one section each week.

Our goal in writing this book is to take the clinical "gold standards" of care for asthma and break them down into useful, straightforward steps to assist you in successfully caring for your child. We hope that you and your child enjoy Zoey's journey through the zones.

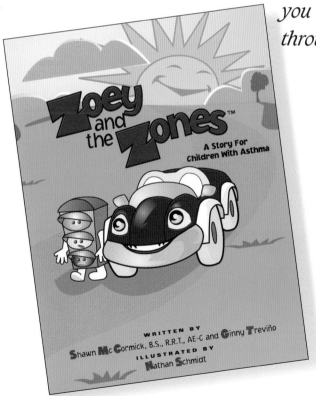

To Order your copy of:

Zoey and the Zones™
A Story for Children with Asthma

by phone call toll-free:
1-866-ASK-ZOEY
on the web:
www.zoeyzones.com

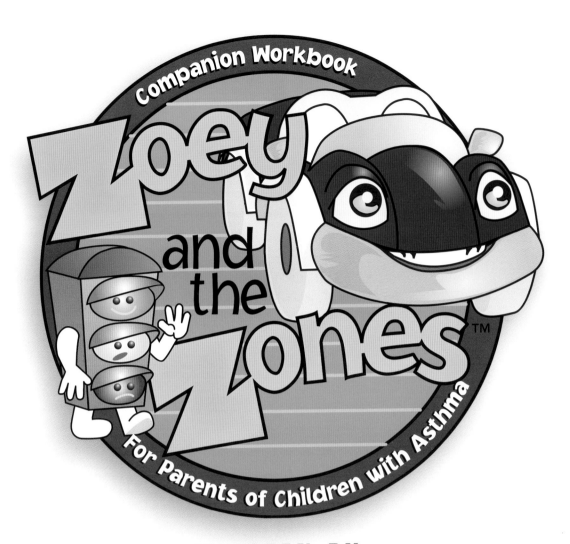

Companion Workbook

Zoey and the Zones™

For Parents of Children with Asthma

WRITTEN BY

Shawn McCormick, B.S., R.R.T., AE-C
and Ginny Treviño

ILLUSTRATIONS BY

Nathan Schmidt

LAYOUT AND DESIGN BY

Pamela Schmidt, Thumbnails

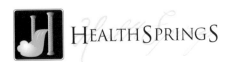

HealthSprings

The principles and guidelines used in the workbook were derived from the National Institutes of Health (NIH), which have set the "gold standards" for physicians and other clinicians to use in caring for patients with asthma. The eleven sections of the workbook have been designed as an educational journey for parents of children with asthma.

At the end of each section are children's activities which will help your child learn the basic information provided in the parent pages. You should plan to work with your child through the activities to ensure that they understand the concepts. We recommend that you work through the book at a pace that is comfortable for both you and your child. Completing one new section each week works well for many families.

The two major NIH standards used for the basis of this workbook are the peak flow monitor and the "zone" plans. Although the workbook addresses all aspects of managing asthma, these two standards are the foundation of understanding when an asthma patient is getting into trouble and how to identify and take action to stop an impending attack or "episode."

Zoey will take your child on an entertaining and educational journey through the asthma zones. The zones are color coded green, yellow, and red. They mirror a traffic light in their significance.

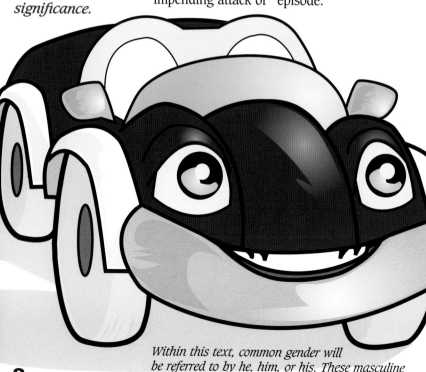

Within this text, common gender will be referred to by he, him, or his. These masculine pronouns include both male and female.

ZOEY AND LIGHT BUDDY WILL TEACH YOU AND YOUR CHILD THE SKILLS YOU NEED TO SUCCESSFULLY MANAGE ASTHMA.

THIS INCLUDES:

- A basic understanding of the disease asthma.
- A basic understanding of medications used to treat asthma and the importance of taking medications properly, depending upon your child's current zone.
- A clear understanding of how your child's peak flow and asthma symptoms correlate with the three asthma zones.
- Proper use of the peak flow meter, metered dose inhalers (MDI's), spacers, and nebulizer compressor.
- Identifying and lessening environmental "triggers" that may be causing asthma episodes in your child's home and school.
- A basic understanding of the importance of exercise and how to lessen asthma symptoms with exercise.
- A basic understanding of proper nutrition for children with asthma.
- A basic understanding of how to relax and minimize "panic" during an asthma episode.
- An understanding of various resources available for children with asthma and their families.

*P*rogressing through the workbook will help you and your child grasp the basic knowledge needed to manage asthma and decrease the frequency and severity of attacks or episodes. Each section will include Parent Pages and related activities for your child.

It is also an invaluable guide to give you the tools you need to help your child with this chronic illness. For best results, we recommend you and your child go through this workbook together and seek professional help with questions from your doctor or asthma educator.

It is important to remember that any person with a chronic illness needs to be seen on a regular basis by a doctor who is qualified to manage their particular disease.

Questions and concerns about specific medications and treatments for the illness should always be discussed with the doctor.

We hope this workbook assists you in answering your questions about asthma. We also hope that Zoey brings your child thoughtful entertainment.

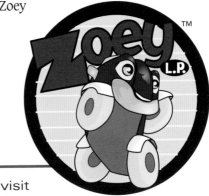

For more information about asthma and Zoey, please visit our Website at **www.zoeyzones.com** or call our toll-free hotline at **1-866-ASK-ZOEY.**

PARENT PAGE - SECTION I

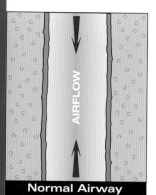

Normal Airway

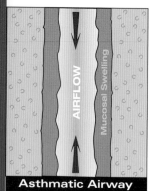

Asthmatic Airway

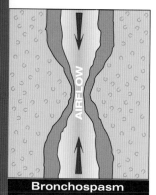

Bronchospasm

Common Asthma Symptoms

- *wheezing*
- *coughing*
- *shortness of breath*
- *chest tightness*
- *fatigue*

WHAT IS ASTHMA?

Asthma is a chronic disease that inflames the airways in your child's lungs. This means that his airways are swollen and sensitive. The swelling is **always there**, even when your child feels good. The swelling can be controlled with medicine and by staying away from things that irritate your child's airways. In addition to being swollen, the airways sometimes spasm and narrow, causing bronchospasm. This results in an asthma attack which is characterized by wheezing, coughing, or shortness of breath. For a long time, people believed that the airway was normal between bronchospasms, but we now know this isn't true. The swelling never goes away, even though it can be controlled. The bottom line is that to control asthma, you have to control the swelling and treat the bronchospasm when it occurs.

WHAT CAUSES ASTHMA?

The basic cause of asthma is not known. There are many theories being researched at this time by doctors and scientists. They still don't have an answer to why some people get asthma and others do not. They do know that it can run in families. Later in the book, you will be asked a series of questions to determine if this disease affects other members of your family.

Asthma attacks, also known as flare-ups, exacerbations, or episodes, can be caused by a variety of "triggers." Eighty percent of children with asthma have allergies to various dander, dust, mold, or pollens. If your child has been diagnosed with asthma, it may be beneficial to have him tested by an allergist to identify his specific allergies or sensitivities. You need to discuss this option with your child's doctor.

Other children have exercise-induced asthma. This means that they may experience coughing, wheezing, or excessive fatigue when they play, participate in sports, or exercise. If your child complains of these types of symptoms, or they are reported by your child's teacher or coach, you should inform your doctor. He may need to perform a Pulmonary Function Test in conjunction with exercise to determine if your child has exercise-induced asthma. A Pulmonary Function Test is a non-invasive, painless procedure that typically can be performed on children five years and older. The Pulmonary Function Test is often performed in your doctor's office and is usually covered by insurance companies.

WHAT ARE COMMON TRIGGERS?

All types of asthma have triggers that lead to attacks. Part of this workbook will teach you and your child to identify the triggers that cause your child's attacks. Some of the more common triggers are:

- Molds and pollens
- Dust
- Dander or flakes from the skin, hair, or feathers of pets
- Cockroaches
- Cigarette and wood smoke
- Upper respiratory infections such as cold and flu
- Scented products such as hairspray, perfume, cosmetics, potpourri, scented candles, incense, air and carpet fresheners
- Air pollution
- Strong odors or fumes from fresh paint, cleaning products, laundry products, cooking and automobile fumes
- Food sensitivities: e.g., shrimp, peanuts, olives, dried fruit
- Some medications such as aspirin and beta-blockers
- Stress, anxiety, fear, and depression
- Changes in the weather or temperature

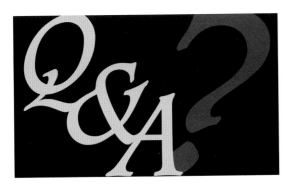

HOW IS ASTHMA DIAGNOSED?

A parent is usually the first person to recognize when their child has a breathing problem. A combination of information leads doctors to the diagnosis of asthma. This includes family history of asthma, symptoms that your child has, and lung study tests. The Pulmonary Function Test (PFT) is an important tool in diagnosing asthma in children five years and older; however, some children cannot perform the maneuver adequately until after age seven. Specifically, doctors evaluate your child's FEV1 value compared to the normal value for your child's age, sex, race, height, and weight. This result, along with the history and symptoms associated with your child's illness, helps determine if your child will be diagnosed with this chronic illness. Peak flow information is very valuable for the ongoing monitoring of your child's asthma; however, it is not usually used in the diagnosis of the disease.

The FEV1 is the amount of air that your child can forcefully exhale in 1 second. Because asthma is considered an obstructive airway disease, the speed at which your child can exhale is usually slower than normal. When your child has a PFT performed, and the FEV1 is lower than normal, your child will be given a bronchodilator treatment before having the PFT performed again. An improved FEV1 performance, after taking a bronchodilator treatment, is a strong indicator that your child has asthma.

CAN ASTHMA BE CURED?

Asthma cannot be cured, but it can be treated and controlled. Your child can become free of symptoms all or most of the time, but asthma does not go away when your child's symptoms go away. You and your child must always take care of his asthma.

As your child grows older, the asthma may change. It could get better or worse, requiring more or less medicine. This is why it is important to see a doctor on a regular basis for the management of this chronic disease.

HOW IS ASTHMA CONTROLLED?

You and your child play the biggest role in taking care of the asthma. These are your jobs:

- Take medicines as prescribed by your child's doctor. Be compliant with your asthma treatment plan.
- Monitor peak flow on a routine basis.
- Recognize the onset of symptoms that lead to asthma attacks and act quickly to stop the attack.
- Keep your child away from triggers that lead to an asthma attack.
- Ask your child's doctor or asthma educator all questions or concerns that you have regarding the disease.
- See your child's doctor at least every six months or more frequently if needed.

WHAT CAN BE EXPECTED FROM PROPER ASTHMA TREATMENT?

You and your child should expect to live free of asthma symptoms all or most of the time. Your child can learn to be active in sports and exercise without symptoms, sleep throughout the night without symptoms, prevent asthma attacks, avoid side effects from asthma medicines, and have lungs that work well. Zoey will teach you and your child how to gain the skills and confidence needed to live and achieve these goals.

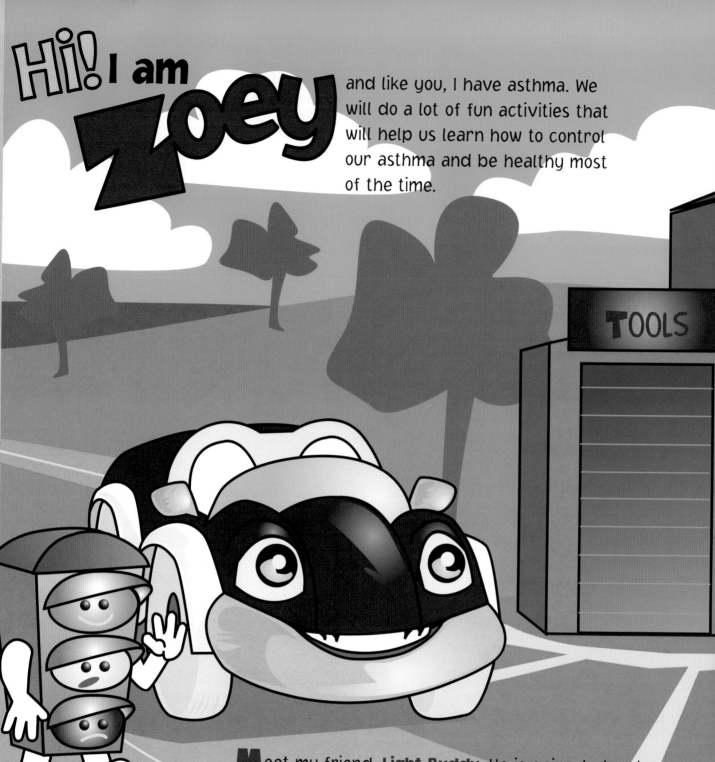

Hi! I am Zoey

and like you, I have asthma. We will do a lot of fun activities that will help us learn how to control our asthma and be healthy most of the time.

TOOLS

Meet my friend, **Light Buddy.** He is going to teach us about **The Zones**. They are like a traffic light—Red, Yellow, and Green.

Lets get ready to go! Follow me...

What is Asthma?

Inside your lungs there are little tubes called airways.

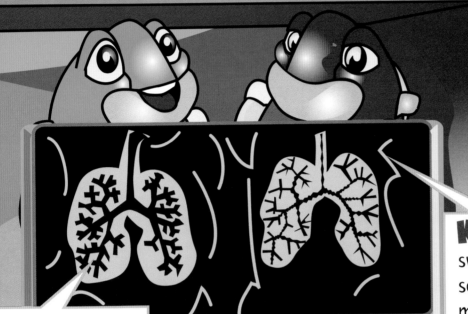

Kids who don't have asthma have airways that are smooth and wide inside.

Kids with asthma have swollen airways that are sometimes narrow. This makes them cough, wheeze, or feel short of breath. A doctor may give them medicine to open the tubes in their lungs so that it is easier to breathe.

Can you find these words...

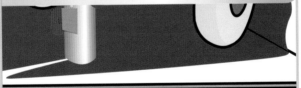

L	A	Z	Z	N	S	Q	D	M	R
T	U	O	R	Y	P	A	J	E	O
D	E	N	W	J	I	T	D	D	T
Y	Y	E	G	R	H	T	Z	I	C
A	L	S	W	S	N	I	Y	C	O
P	E	A	K	F	L	O	W	I	D
U	Y	A	M	H	T	S	A	N	J
S	O	P	T	R	I	G	G	E	R
A	T	T	A	C	K	S	O	O	X
A	K	V	V	I	V	Z	K	V	V

ASTHMA	MEDICINE
AIRWAYS	TRIGGER
DOCTOR	LUNGS
ATTACK	ZOEY
PEAK FLOW	ZONES

7

Section I Summary

SECTION 1 - INTRODUCTION

1. What is Asthma?

    Asthma is a chronic respiratory disease that is characterized by inflammation inside the airways and periodic constriction or bronchospasm of the outer walls of the airways.

2. What information is used to diagnose asthma?
- A family history of asthma
- Pulmonary function tests
- Asthma Symptoms

3. What are the most common symptoms of asthma?
- Wheezing
- Coughing
- Shortness of breath
- Tightness in chest

4. What are the most common triggers for asthma attacks?
- Molds and pollens
- Dust
- Animal dander
- Cockroaches
- Cigarette and wood smoke
- Upper respiratory infections
- Scented products
- Air pollution

5. There is NO cure for asthma.

6. With proper management, your child can expect to live free of asthma symptoms all or most of the time.

7. The following activities will help you and your child gain control over asthma:
- Monitoring peak flow regularly.
- Recognizing the onset of asthma symptoms and using the zone treatment plan.
- Taking medicines as prescribed by your child's doctor.
- Keeping regular doctor's appointments.
- Asking the doctor or asthma educator questions about the disease and proper management.

NOTES

_____

_____

_____

_____

_____

Asthma Severity

*T*he National Institutes of Health have established four classes of asthma severity: mild intermittent, mild persistent, moderate persistent, and severe persistent. This classification system shows the severity of your child's asthma. Although this classification is important in developing the treatment plan, you need to remember that **all asthma is serious** and your child may experience extreme attacks, even if he has a mild classification.

Although many children experience different levels of severity during an asthma attack, their disease falls into one severity classification. These classifications are determined before treatment. In other words, you need to think about how your child's asthma was before he was diagnosed and started on asthma medicine. On the next few pages, Zoey will guide you and your child through a series of questions that will help you determine your child's asthma severity. The questions will be geared toward your child's daytime and nighttime symptoms, and the results of his pulmonary function tests. Remember that asthma symptoms are not the same for all children. Some may experience wheezing, others coughing, shortness of breath, or a tight feeling in their chest. Many children have a combination of these symptoms. Nighttime symptoms mean that the symptoms described above, wheezing, coughing, shortness of breath, or chest tightness occur at nighttime and wake your child up. Earlier in the workbook we discussed pulmonary function testing and how the FEV1 is used to diagnose asthma. To determine your child's asthma severity classification, you will need to get this result from your child's doctor.

MILD INTERMITTENT ASTHMA

Mild intermittent asthma means your child has periodic asthma that is generally mild, although the attacks may sometimes be intense. It is characterized by the following:

1) Wheezing, coughing, shortness of breath, or chest tightness that occurs twice per week or less.

2) There may be no symptoms and normal peak flows between asthma attacks.

3) Asthma attacks are usually infrequent and/or brief.

4) Your child is awakened during the night by wheezing, coughing, shortness of breath, or chest tightness less than two times per month.

5) Your child's FEV1 on the pulmonary function test is greater than or equal to 80% of predicted measurements for your child's age, sex, race, height, and weight.

ASTHMA SEVERITY

MILD Intermittent

MILD Persistent

MODERATE Persistent

SEVERE Persistent

MILD PERSISTENT ASTHMA

Mild persistent asthma means your child's asthma is still considered mild, but is always present. It is characterized by the following:

1) Wheezing, coughing, shortness of breath, or chest tightness occurs more than twice per week but less than once per day.

2) Asthma attacks affect your child's physical activities (playing, exercising, or participating in school PE, or sports).

3) Asthma attacks occur more than two times per week, but less than once per day.

4) Your child is awakened during the night by wheezing, coughing, shortness of breath, or chest tightness three to four times per month.

5) Your child's FEV1 on the pulmonary function test is greater than or equal to 80% of predicted measurements for your child's age, sex, race, height, and weight.

MODERATE PERSISTENT ASTHMA

Moderate persistent asthma means your child has daily symptoms and frequent asthma attacks. It is characterized by the following:

1) Daily wheezing, coughing, shortness of breath, or chest tightness.

2) Asthma attacks affect your child's physical activities (playing, exercising, participating in school PE, or sports).

3) Asthma attacks occur at least twice per week.

4) Your child is awakened during the night by wheezing, coughing, shortness of breath, or chest tightness more than once per week.

5) Your child's FEV1 on the pulmonary function test is between 60% and 80% of predicted measurement for your child's age, sex, race, height, and weight.

SEVERE PERSISTENT ASTHMA

Severe persistent asthma means your child has continuous symptoms, awakens frequently during the night, and has frequent asthma attacks. It is characterized by the following:

1) Continuous wheezing, coughing, shortness of breath, or chest tightness.

2) Your child has very limited physical activity (unable to play, exercise, or participate in school PE, or sports).

3) Your child has frequent asthma attacks.

4) Your child is frequently awakened during the night with wheezing, coughing, shortness of breath, or chest tightness.

5) Your child's FEV1 on the pulmonary function test is less than or equal to 60% of predicted measurement for your child's age, sex, race, height, and weight.

As you think about your child and identify his category, it is important to remember that you are classifying your child's asthma *before* treatment began. Even if your child falls into the mild categories, he may still experience attacks that can be severe and life threatening. Because of this possible severity, you must learn how to identify when your child is getting into trouble. This includes the steps to take to treat an attack and how to avoid the triggers that may lead to an attack in your child.

On the next few pages, Zoey will be asking you and your child a series of questions about his asthma. Your child will need your help to answer these questions. Use the answers to determine his asthma classification. As always, ask your doctor or asthma educator for assistance with any question that you and your child might have about asthma classification.

Parents Medical History Questionnaire

	YES	NO
1. Do you, your parents, or other children have asthma? If yes, please list: 		
2. Does your child make wheezing or whistling sounds when he breathes?		
3. Does your child cough a lot?		
4. Does your child cough at night?		
5. Do asthma symptoms awaken your child at night?		
6. Does your child complain of chest tightness or a "squeezing" feeling?		
7. Does your child breathe better after he takes his medicine?		

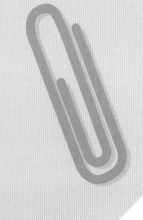

How Bad Is My Asthma?

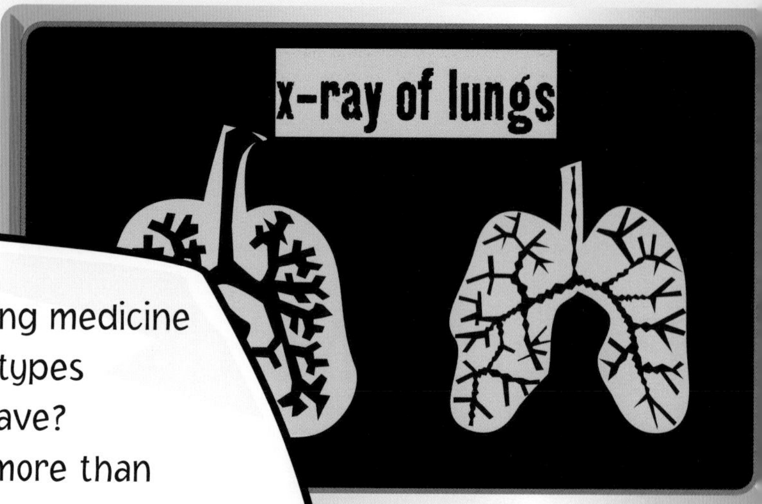

x-ray of lungs

1) Before you started taking medicine for your asthma, what types of symptoms did you have? (You may have had more than one of these symptoms. Check all of them that you had).

❑ Wheezing

❑ Coughing

❑ Shortness of breath

❑ Tightness in chest

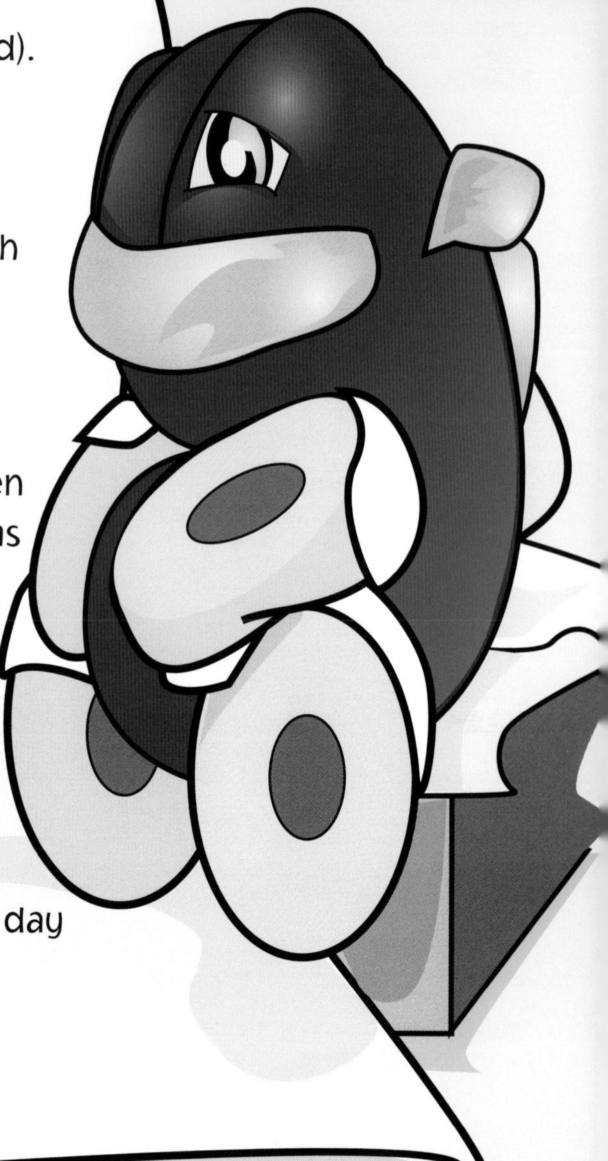

2) Before you started your asthma medicine, how often did you have the symptoms that you checked above?

❑ Two times or less per week

❑ More than two times per week, but less than once per day

❑ Every day

❑ All of the time

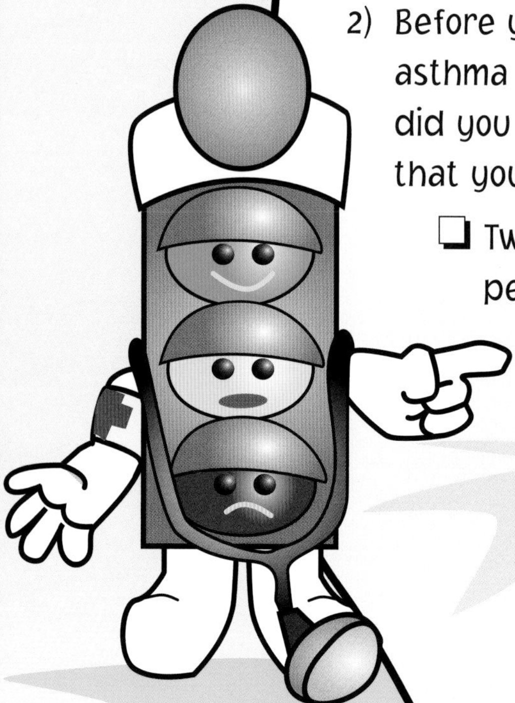

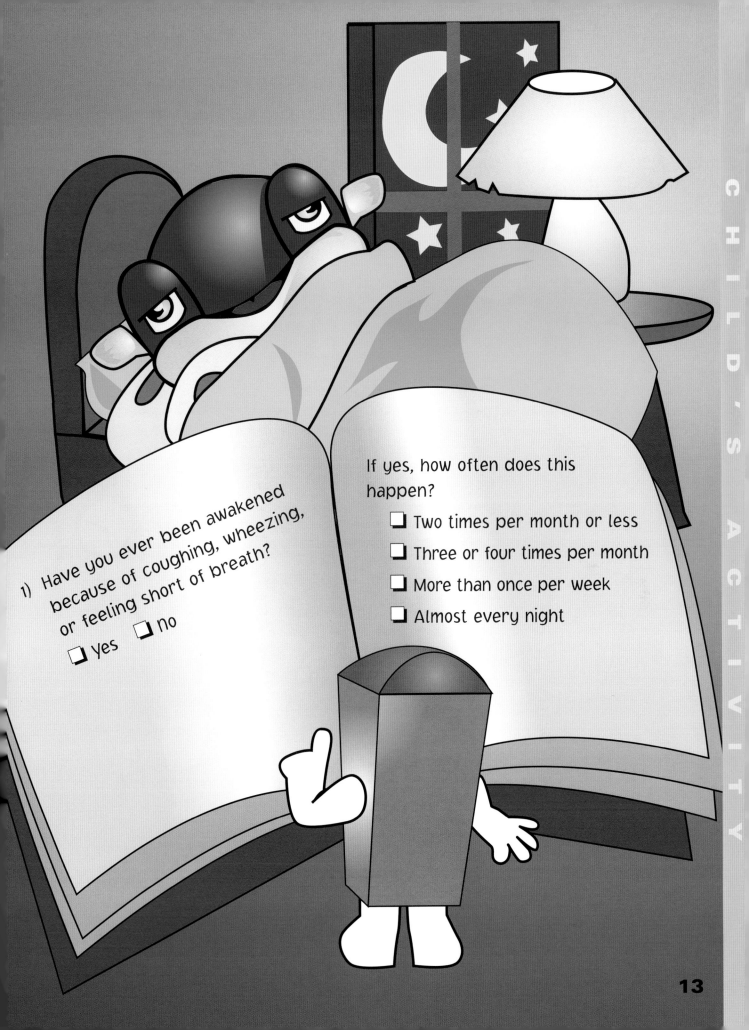

1) Have you ever been awakened because of coughing, wheezing, or feeling short of breath?

☐ Yes ☐ No

If yes, how often does this happen?

☐ Two times per month or less

☐ Three or four times per month

☐ More than once per week

☐ Almost every night

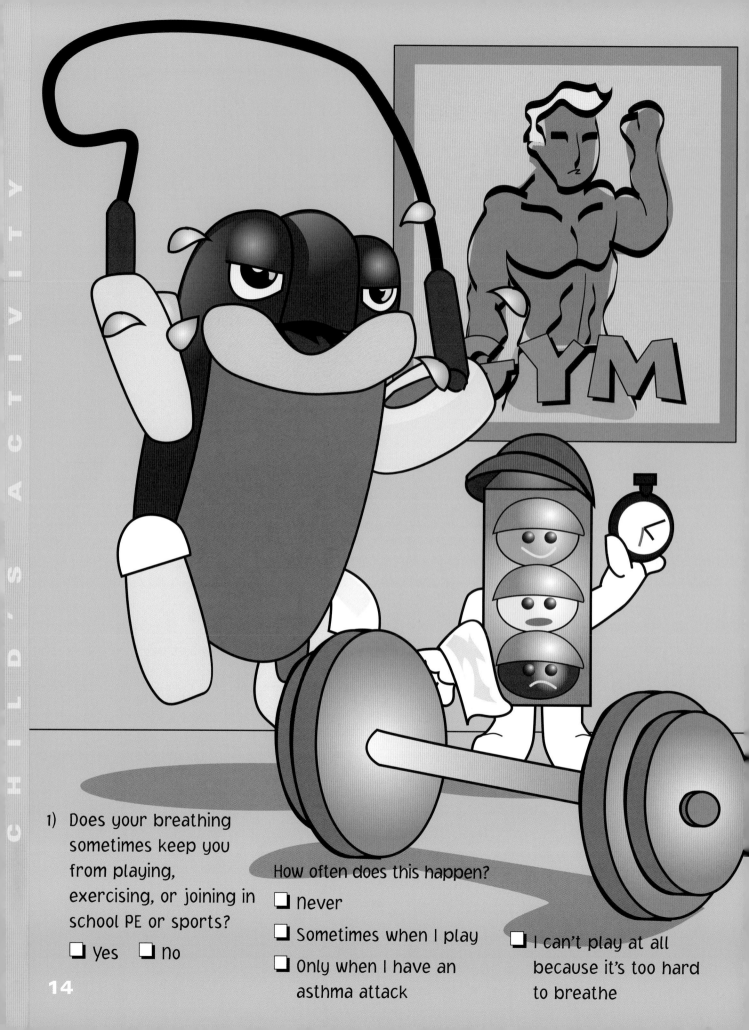

1) Does your breathing sometimes keep you from playing, exercising, or joining in school PE or sports?

❑ Yes ❑ No

How often does this happen?

❑ Never

❑ Sometimes when I play

❑ Only when I have an asthma attack

❑ I can't play at all because it's too hard to breathe

14

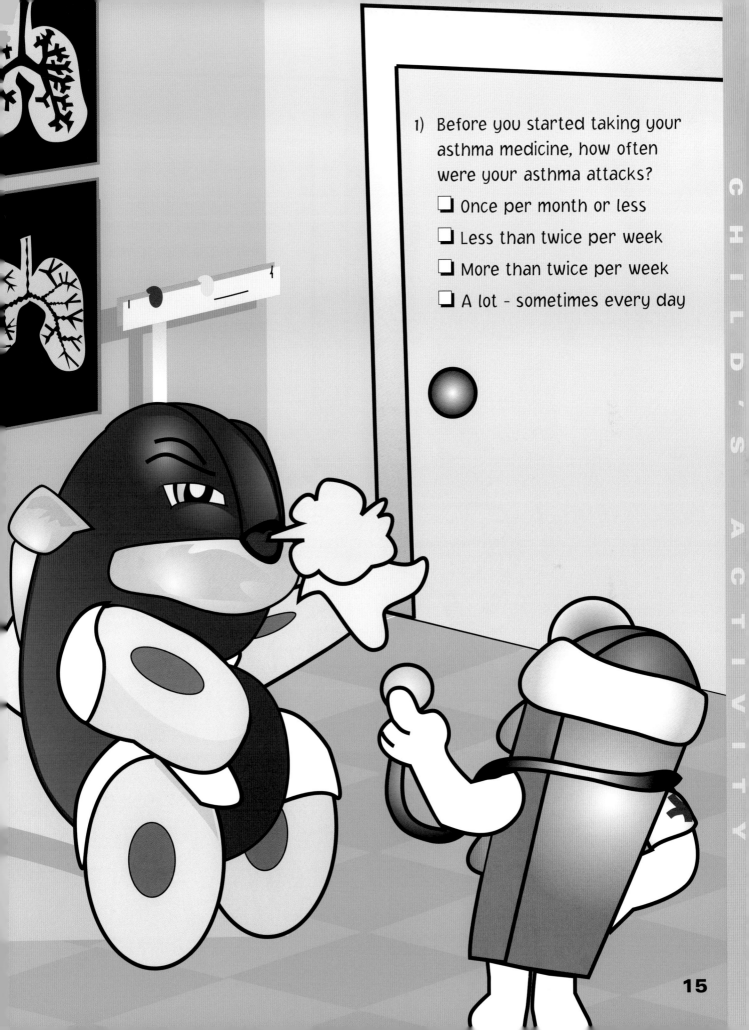

1) Before you started taking your asthma medicine, how often were your asthma attacks?
   ☐ Once per month or less
   ☐ Less than twice per week
   ☐ More than twice per week
   ☐ A lot – sometimes every day

15

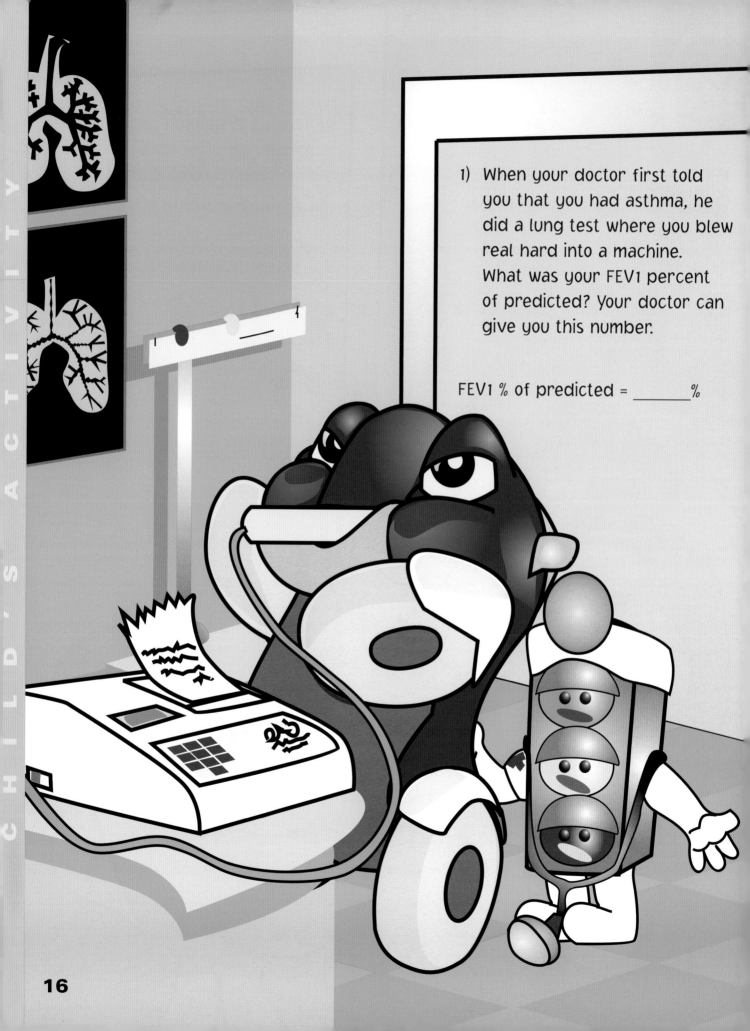

1) When your doctor first told you that you had asthma, he did a lung test where you blew real hard into a machine. What was your FEV1 percent of predicted? Your doctor can give you this number.

FEV1 % of predicted = _____%

Asthma Severity Chart

Asthma	Symptoms	Nighttime Symptoms	Attacks	Activity	FEV1
Mild Intermittent	Less than 2/week No symptoms between attacks	Less than 2/month	Infrequent and/or brief	Normal	At or above 80%
Mild Persistent	More than 2/week but less than 1/day	3 to 4 per month	Less than 2/week	Decreased with attacks	At or above 80%
Moderate Persistent	Daily	More than 1/week	More than 2/week	Decreased with attacks	Between 60%-80%
Severe Persistent	Continuous	Often	Daily or often	Unable to play	Less than 60%

Check your answers on pages 12 through 16 to see how bad your asthma is:

I have _____ asthma.

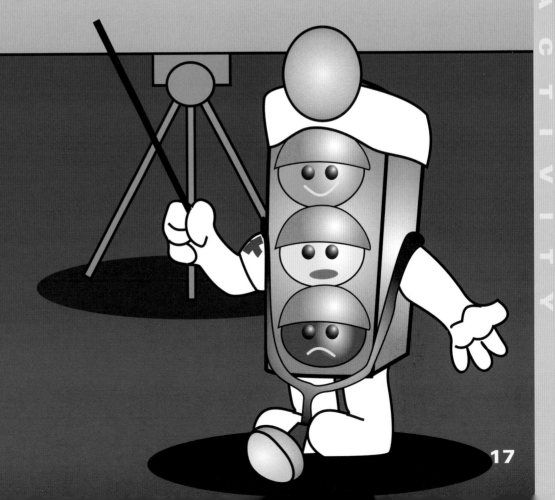

Section II Summary

SECTION II - ASTHMA SEVERITY

1. All classifications of asthma are serious.

2. Children with any of the severity classifications, even "mild," can have serious or life-threatening attacks.

NOTES

_____

_____

_____

_____

_____

_____

_____

_____

_____

_____

_____

_____

_____

The Zones

NOW THAT YOUR CHILD'S ASTHMA HAS BEEN CLASSIFIED AND YOU RECOGNIZE YOUR CHILD'S ASTHMA SYMPTOMS, WE WILL MOVE INTO A MORE DETAILED EXPLANATION OF THE ASTHMA ZONES.

Regardless of your child's classification, you must learn the characteristics of each zone. All asthmatics experience episodes that result from an escalation of symptoms. The zones help identify how bad your child's attack is and what action should be taken for relief and recovery.

The NIH has established the zones for guiding treatment based on asthma symptoms and lung performance. They are recognized by all caregivers as the standard treatment plans for all classifications of asthma. There are three components to the zone treatment plans. They are:

1. Identifying escalating symptoms.
2. Tracking peak flow results.
3. Adherence to medication regimens.

The next section of the workbook explains peak flow monitoring. You and your child must master the technique for peak flow monitoring because it is the basis for identifying what zone your child is in at any given time.

The color coded zones were developed because of their simplicity and their correlation to the colors of a traffic light.

GREEN ZONE

This zone reflects times when your child's asthma is under control, peak flows are **within 80%** of his personal best, and he is having no symptoms. This represents "go" in an asthma child's life.

YELLOW ZONE

This zone represents a "caution" period for your child. His peak flow is **between 50%-80%** of his personal best, and he is experiencing symptoms associated with an asthma attack. The symptoms may be coughing, wheezing, and some mild shortness of breath. You and your child will learn to identify when he is entering this zone, what to do, and how to get him back into the green zone.

RED ZONE

The color red on a traffic light signals "*STOP!*". As with the traffic light, the red zone in asthma means stop and signals a medical emergency. The peak flow is **below 50%** of your child's personal best and he is experiencing a full-blown asthma episode, usually with wheezing and/or coughing, and shortness of breath. Zoey will explain what emergency steps to take when your child is in the red zone, and how to avoid getting to this point.

19

Zones

There are three Asthma Zones, Green, Yellow, and Red, just like a traffic light.

Draw a line from the following words to the correct light.

Caution

Red

Green

Stop

Yellow

Go

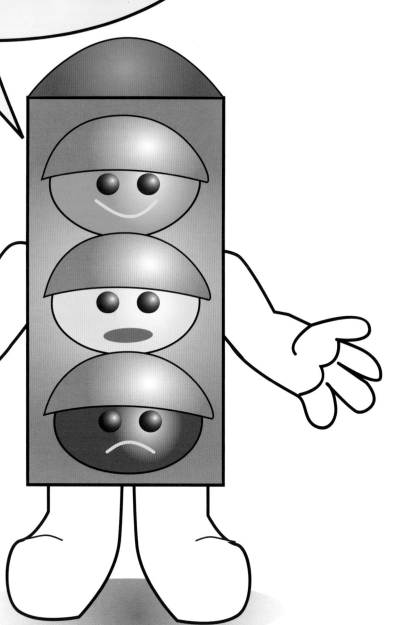

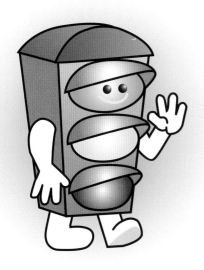

Green Zone:

Go
No Asthma Symptoms

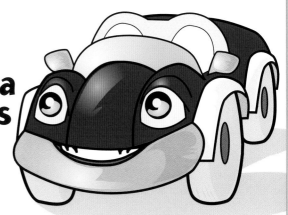

Yellow Zone:

Caution
Having asthma symptoms
Feeling yucky

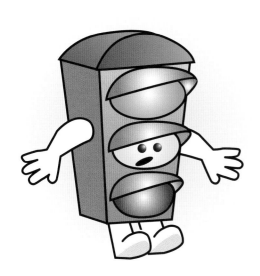

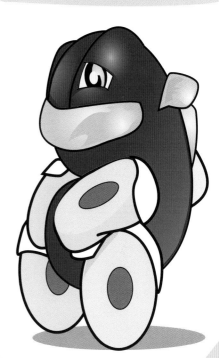

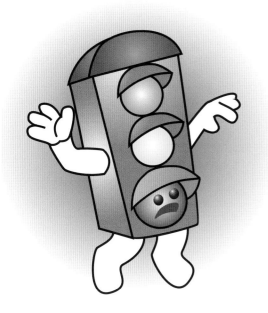

Red Zone:

Stop
Breathing is hard

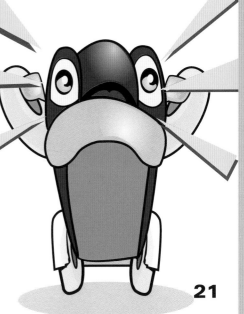

Section III Summary

SECTION III - THE ZONES

1. The three asthma zones are:

- Green
- Yellow
- Red

2. The major components of the asthma zone treatment plan include:

- Tracking peak flow results.
- Adhering to medication regimens.
- Identifying and responding to escalating asthma symptoms.

NOTES

_____

_____

_____

_____

_____

_____

_____

_____

_____

_____

_____

_____

PEAK FLOW METERS

A peak flow meter is a small, inexpensive device, used to see how well your child's air moves out of his lungs. There are many types and brands of peak flow meters available. Our recommendation is to find one that's small, compact, and easy for you and your child to use and read.

Two commonly used meters are the Asthma Mentor and the Personal Best, made by Respironics. However, check with your doctor for his or her recommendations.

When your child has an asthma attack, the airway spasms and narrows. As a result, the peak flow reading goes down. This may happen hours or even days before your child begins to have asthma symptoms. By monitoring your child's peak flow daily, you will learn to identify when your child is getting into trouble and how to stop the onset of a full-blown asthma attack. The daily use of a peak flow meter will also help you and your child's doctor learn what makes the asthma worse, when to add or stop medicines, and when to get emergency treatment.

Children with any persistent classification of asthma should use peak flow meters. They are normally recommended for children ages five years and older. Children younger than five may have difficulty performing the technique needed for an accurate reading. Because every child is different, it is necessary to establish your child's "personal best" peak flow reading. All of the zone treatment plans are based on your child's personal best peak flow result.

To determine your child's personal best peak flow number, you must take and record the readings daily for three weeks, preferably in the early afternoon each day. The peak flow meter should be used before your child uses his bronchodilator (albuterol), if prescribed by the doctor.

Remember, peak flow monitoring is not a treatment for asthma! It is simply a tool used to track how well air moves out of the lungs so that you and your child can identify when he is getting into trouble and what steps to take to stop an asthma attack. By recording your child's peak flow results on a daily basis, your child will get into the habit of performing this test routinely. It is important to create a diary that will become a routine part of your child's asthma treatment plan. This diary will also give your child's doctor important information. Always take it with you when your child visits the doctor for any reason.

> *It is important for the peak flow meter test to become a routine part of your child's asthma treatment plan. This reading identifies what Zone your child is in.*

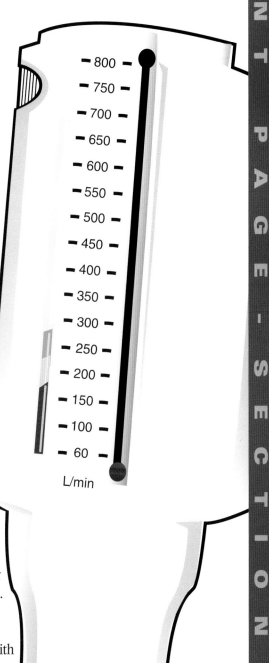

800
750
700
650
600
550
500
450
400
350
300
250
200
150
100
60
L/min

23

Peak Flows

A peak flow meter is a tool that is easy to use and doesn't hurt. Zoey uses his peak flow meter every day to check his lungs. Zoey and your parents will help you find your best number. The bigger the number, the better your lungs are doing. When your peak flow number gets smaller, it means your asthma is getting worse. Zoey will show you things to do to make you feel better and stop an asthma attack.

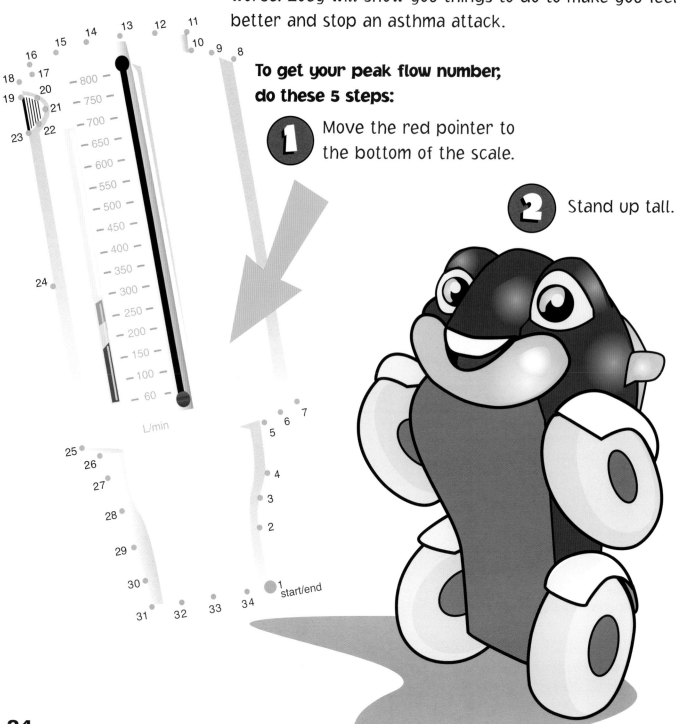

To get your peak flow number, do these 5 steps:

1 Move the red pointer to the bottom of the scale.

2 Stand up tall.

L/min

start/end

IMPORTANT: For complete information, refer to the device instructions.

CHILD'S ACTIVITY

3 Take a deep breath, fill up your lungs, and hold your breath.

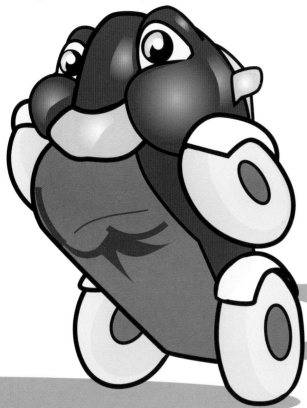

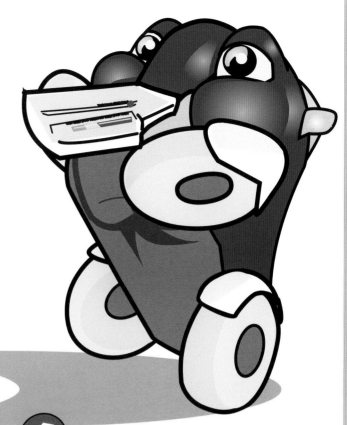

4 Put the meter in your mouth and close your lips around it. Do not put your tongue inside the meter.

5 Blow out as hard and fast as you can, in one blow.

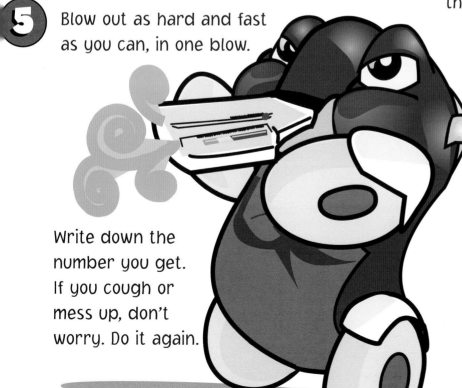

Write down the number you get. If you cough or mess up, don't worry. Do it again.

Repeat steps 1-5 two more times. Write down the biggest number of the three tries in your diary.

Initial Peak Flow Diary

	Date	Your Best Number	How Do I Feel Today	Meds Used
1			Great / Not So Good / Yucky	Yes / No
2			Great / Not So Good / Yucky	Yes / No
3			Great / Not So Good / Yucky	Yes / No
4			Great / Not So Good / Yucky	Yes / No
5			Great / Not So Good / Yucky	Yes / No
6			Great / Not So Good / Yucky	Yes / No
7			Great / Not So Good / Yucky	Yes / No
8			Great / Not So Good / Yucky	Yes / No
9			Great / Not So Good / Yucky	Yes / No
10			Great / Not So Good / Yucky	Yes / No
11			Great / Not So Good / Yucky	Yes / No
12			Great / Not So Good / Yucky	Yes / No
13			Great / Not So Good / Yucky	Yes / No
14			Great / Not So Good / Yucky	Yes / No
15			Great / Not So Good / Yucky	Yes / No
16			Great / Not So Good / Yucky	Yes / No
17			Great / Not So Good / Yucky	Yes / No
18			Great / Not So Good / Yucky	Yes / No
19			Great / Not So Good / Yucky	Yes / No
20			Great / Not So Good / Yucky	Yes / No
21			Great / Not So Good / Yucky	Yes / No

Can you find your best number?
Write it here

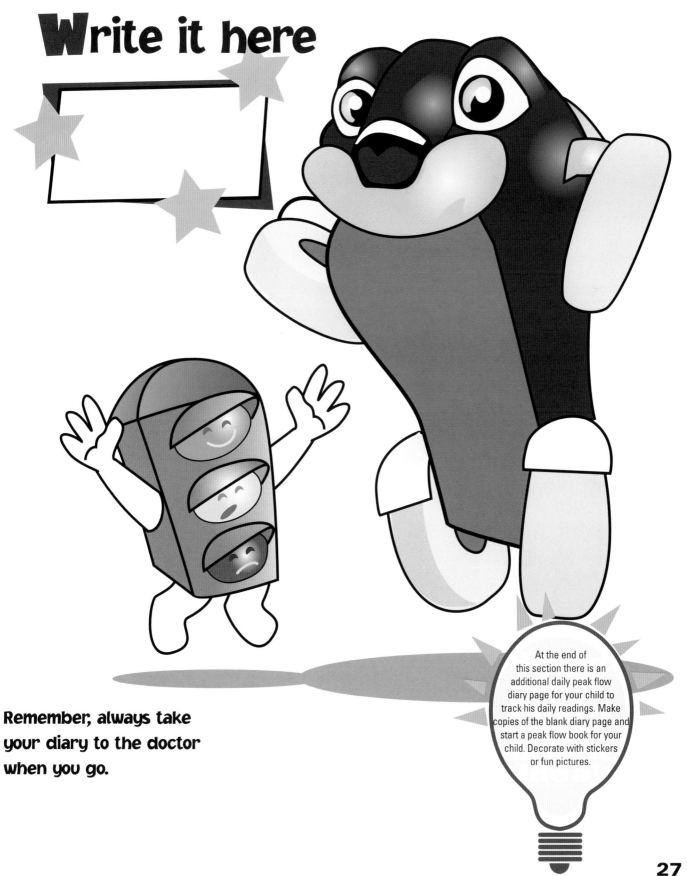

Remember, always take your diary to the doctor when you go.

At the end of this section there is an additional daily peak flow diary page for your child to track his daily readings. Make copies of the blank diary page and start a peak flow book for your child. Decorate with stickers or fun pictures.

Zoey's Zones

Green Zone = **Peak Flow is > 80% of personal best**

Yellow Zone = **Peak Flow is between 50% – 80% of personal best**

Red Zone = **Peak Flow is < 50% of personal best**

Zoey's Zone Chart

Zoey's Personal Best Peak Flow is 400

Zoey's Green Zone =

GO — Peak Flow greater than 320

No symptoms

Zoey's Yellow Zone =

Caution — Peak Flow between 200 & 320

Having symptoms, Feeling yucky

Zoey's Red Zone =

Stop — Peak Flow less than 200

Breathing is hard

CHILD'S ACTIVITY

What Zone is Zoey in?

Using Zoey's Zone chart on page 28, color in the right color light on Light Buddy for each Zone Zoey is in.

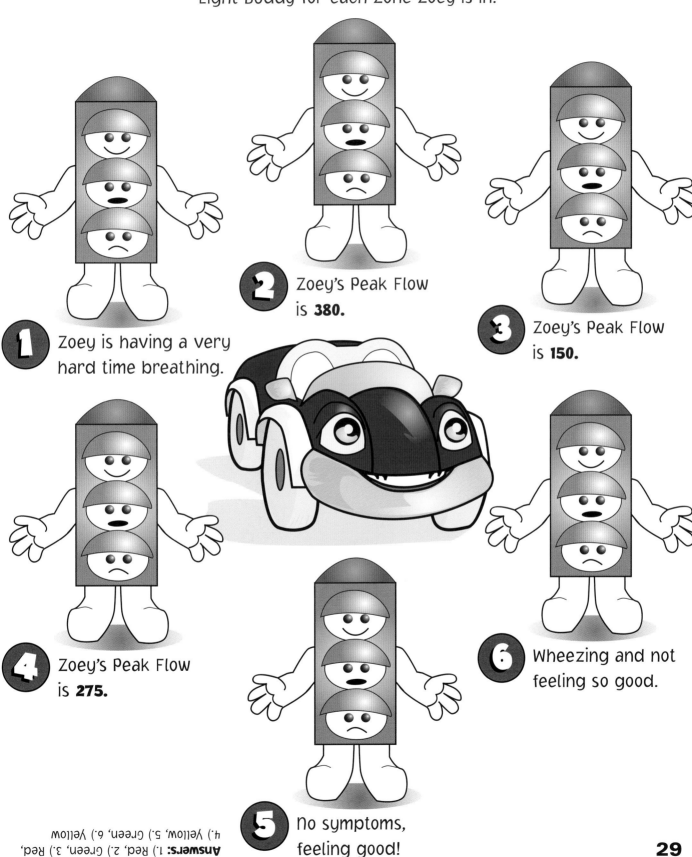

1 Zoey is having a very hard time breathing.

2 Zoey's Peak Flow is **380.**

3 Zoey's Peak Flow is **150.**

4 Zoey's Peak Flow is **275.**

5 No symptoms, feeling good!

6 Wheezing and not feeling so good.

Answers: 1.) Red, 2.) Green, 3.) Red, 4.) Yellow, 5.) Green, 6.) Yellow

Daily Peak Flow Diary

Date	Your Best Number	How Do I Feel Today?	Meds Used
1		Great / Not So Good / Yucky	Yes / No
2		Great / Not So Good / Yucky	Yes / No
3		Great / Not So Good / Yucky	Yes / No
4		Great / Not So Good / Yucky	Yes / No
5		Great / Not So Good / Yucky	Yes / No
6		Great / Not So Good / Yucky	Yes / No
7		Great / Not So Good / Yucky	Yes / No
8		Great / Not So Good / Yucky	Yes / No
9		Great / Not So Good / Yucky	Yes / No
10		Great / Not So Good / Yucky	Yes / No
11		Great / Not So Good / Yucky	Yes / No
12		Great / Not So Good / Yucky	Yes / No
13		Great / Not So Good / Yucky	Yes / No
14		Great / Not So Good / Yucky	Yes / No
15		Great / Not So Good / Yucky	Yes / No
16		Great / Not So Good / Yucky	Yes / No
17		Great / Not So Good / Yucky	Yes / No
18		Great / Not So Good / Yucky	Yes / No
19		Great / Not So Good / Yucky	Yes / No
20		Great / Not So Good / Yucky	Yes / No
21		Great / Not So Good / Yucky	Yes / No
22		Great / Not So Good / Yucky	Yes / No
23		Great / Not So Good / Yucky	Yes / No
24		Great / Not So Good / Yucky	Yes / No
25		Great / Not So Good / Yucky	Yes / No
26		Great / Not So Good / Yucky	Yes / No
27		Great / Not So Good / Yucky	Yes / No
28		Great / Not So Good / Yucky	Yes / No
29		Great / Not So Good / Yucky	Yes / No
30		Great / Not So Good / Yucky	Yes / No
31		Great / Not So Good / Yucky	Yes / No

Section IV Summary

SECTION IV - PEAK FLOW METERS

1. Peak flow results are useful in identifying when your child is beginning to have a problem with their breathing.

2. The higher the peak flow number is, the better your child is doing.

3. Your child's personal best peak flow number is obtained by tracking his results daily for three weeks and taking the highest number.

4. The five steps for correctly performing peak flows are:

- Move the red pointer on the peak flow meter to its lowest number at the bottom of the meter.
- Stand up tall.
- Take a deep breath, fill up your lungs, and hold your breath.
- Put the meter in your mouth and close your lips around it. Do not put your tongue inside the meter.
- Blow out as hard and fast as you can in one breath. If you cough, or mess up, repeat the steps listed above.

5. Green Zone (GO) = Peak flow results are greater than 80% of personal best with no asthma symptoms

6. Yellow Zone (CAUTION) = Peak flow results are between 50% and 80% of personal best with some asthma symptoms.

7. Red Zone (STOP!) = Medical emergency. Peak flow results are less than 50% of personal best and breathing is difficult.

NOTES

_____

_____

_____

_____

_____

_____

_____

_____

Environmental Triggers

*T*here are many different environmental irritants or allergens, known as "triggers," that may increase your child's asthma symptoms or cause an asthma attack.

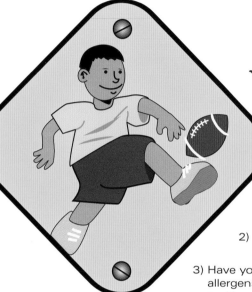

Y*ou now know your child's asthma severity classification. For children with any persistent asthma, it may be necessary to:

1) Identify your child's allergen exposures.

2) Determine if your child has seasonal allergies.

3) Have your child tested for specific allergens that he may be sensitive to. You will need to discuss allergy testing with your child's doctor to determine what type of testing may be done to zero in on specific triggers.

Children with any classification of asthma severity should try to avoid:

1) Exposure to triggers which they are sensitive to.

2) Exposure to tobacco smoke.

3) Outdoor physical activity when air pollution levels are high.

4) Foods containing sulfites.

5) Other foods which they are sensitive to and lead to an asthma attack.

Annual flu vaccines are generally safe, effective, and recommended for children with asthma that are six months of age or older. If you have any questions or concerns about using the vaccine for your child, do not hesitate to ask your child's doctor.

Upper respiratory tract infections are often the number one trigger for asthma attacks in babies and small children. If your child has chronic problems with a runny nose, sinus congestion, coughing, or ear infections, seek advice or treatment from your child's doctor. Left untreated, these illnesses often trigger asthma attacks.

At this point, it is important to begin thinking about possible triggers in your own home that may be causing your child's asthma attacks. On the next two pages there are a series of questions that you need to think about and answer honestly. Although your child may not be sensitive to all of the triggers discussed, you need to take a critical inventory of your own home.

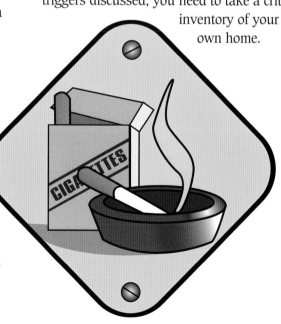

ENVIRONMENTAL QUESTIONNAIRE

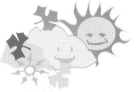

1. Do you have a pet(s) that lives in your house? ❑ yes ❑ no

2. What kind of pet(s) do you have? _____

3. How often do you change your air condition/heating filters? _____

4. What type of flooring do you have throughout most of your home?
    ❑ carpet ❑ linoleum ❑ tile ❑ wood

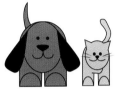

5. What type of flooring is in your child's bedroom?
    ❑ carpet ❑ linoleum ❑ tile ❑ wood

6. How often do you vacuum, sweep, or mop your floors?_____

7. Do you live in a city that has frequent air pollution? ❑ yes ❑ no

8. Do you have any leaky faucets in your home? ❑ yes ❑ no

9. If yes, where are the leaks located? _____

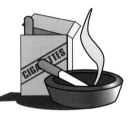

10. When it rains, does your roof leak? ❑ yes ❑ no

11. If yes, what room has leaks?_____

12. If you have a basement, does it sometimes get wet or damp? ❑ yes ❑ no

13. Is there any mold or mildew around your sinks, bathtubs, showers, toilets,
    doors, or windows? ❑ yes ❑ no

14. Do you have cockroaches in your house? ❑ yes ❑ no

15. Does your child seem to wheeze, cough, feel short of breath, or experience
    tightness in his chest more at specific times of the year? ❑ yes ❑ no

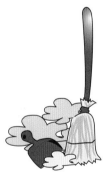

16. If yes, when are your child's asthma symptoms worse?
    ❑ Early Spring (trees)   ❑ Late Spring (grasses)
    ❑ Late Summer to Fall (weeds)   ❑ Summer and Fall (molds)

17. Do you or anyone else in your home smoke? ❑ yes ❑ no

18. Does your child's babysitter or other relatives smoke? ❑ yes ❑ no

19. Do you have a fireplace in your home? ❑ yes ❑ no

20. If yes, does it burn real wood or does it have electric or gas logs?
    ❑ real wood ❑ electrical ❑ gas

Continued on next page

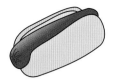

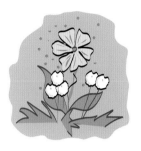

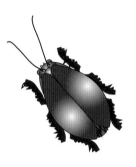

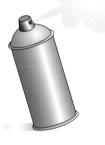

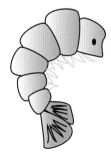

Continued from previous page

21. Do you have a wood burning stove or coal burning stove in your house?
❑ yes ❑ no

22. Do you use kerosene heaters in your house? ❑ yes ❑ no

23. Does perfume or air fresheners make it hard for your child to breathe?
❑ yes ❑ no

24. Do you use scented candles or potpourri in your home? ❑ yes ❑ no

25. Do you use bleach, pine cleaners, ammonia, or other strong smelling agents as cleaning products? ❑ yes ❑ no

26. Does your child often have a runny nose ? ❑ yes ❑ no

27. Is your child's nose often stopped up? ❑ yes ❑ no

28. Does eating any of the following foods make it harder for your child to breathe, or make his throat hurt?
❑ shrimp ❑ dried fruit ❑ hot dogs or bologna ❑ peanuts/peanut butter
❑ Chinese food ❑ instant potatoes ❑ pickles or relish

29. What medicines does your child take regularly?

_____   _____

_____   _____

_____   _____

30. Does your child use eyedrops? ❑ yes ❑ no

31. If yes, what type of eyedrops? _____

32. Does your child ever take aspirin? ❑ yes ❑ no

33. Does your child's asthma ever get worse after taking any medicine, eyedrops or aspirin? ❑ yes ❑ no

34. If yes, which ones make the asthma worse?

_____

Congratulations!

YOU HAVE JUST COMPLETED A VERY IMPORTANT STEP IN IDENTIFYING POTENTIAL ASTHMA TRIGGERS IN YOUR HOME.

The questions have probably given you a pretty good idea of possible irritants that may be triggering asthma attacks in your child. Although this exercise might seem somewhat overwhelming to you, we will now provide you with a common sense approach to minimizing triggers in your child's living environment. As stated earlier, not everything listed on the questionnaire will be a trigger to your child; however, it makes sense to remove as many of the triggers as possible. Most of the ideas we give you are not intended to raise your household expenses. Many of the ideas may even result in overall cost savings.

ANIMAL DANDER

Animals with hair, fur, or feathers have dander. Dander comes from the fur, feather, hair, saliva, urine, and feces of these types of animals. For children with animal dander sensitivity, just being near these animals can trigger an attack. Although the action needed to remove this trigger is obvious, many pets are beloved members of the family, and the choice to find a new home for them is often difficult. If you don't have a dog, cat, hamster, ferret, or other furry or hairy animal, but you would like your child to have a pet, consider fish or even snakes! If your family is unable to give away a pet, at least attempt to:

1) Keep the pet outside or out of your child's bedroom at all times.

2) Bathe the pet weekly. This includes cats!

3) Clean any "accidents" immediately and thoroughly.

4) Empty the cat litter box every two or three days and keep it away from your child's bedroom.

5) Keep pets off upholstered furniture and beds; wherever they may shed their hair.

HOUSE DUST

Everyone has house dust! For anyone with asthma, this dust can trigger an attack. When your child breathes large amounts of dust, his inflamed airways may spasm, and lead to an attack. Dust contains microscopic bugs called mites. You can't see them, but trust us, they are everywhere. Besides the obvious places where you see dust, on tables, bookcases, televisions, etc., dust is in your bedding, pillows, carpet, flooring, stuffed toys, "blankies," air conditioning and heating systems, upholstered furniture, lamp shades, curtains, blinds, and vacuum cleaners. No one will ever win the battle against dust; however, there are things you can do to minimize this asthma trigger.

1) Cover your child's mattress and pillow with a zippered allergen-proof cover. Put your mattress pad and sheet over the protector. Put the pillow case over the pillow protector. These types of protectors may be found in stores that carry sheets or other bedding products.

2) Wash your child's sheets and blankets every week in HOT water. It takes a temperature of 130 degrees to kill dust mites. You might not want to use brightly colored sheets because they often fade in hot water.

3) If your child has a favorite stuffed toy or "blankie," only allow them to sleep with one of these items. Like the bedding, it should be washed weekly in HOT water.

4) The optimal type of flooring would be a hard surface. We do recognize that this is often impossible, especially if you live in rented housing. If you cannot remove carpets or rugs throughout your home, you might wish to remove them from your child's bedroom. If that is not possible, you should try the following:

- Vacuum the rugs or carpets at least twice per week. Do not vacuum rooms with your child present, as the vacuum stirs up a lot of dust. If you have a traditional vacuum cleaner with bags, empty and replace them at least monthly. If possible, you might want to purchase a vacuum cleaner that uses a water collection system or HEPA filter.

- Take small rugs outside and shake them out weekly. If possible, wash them monthly.

5) If you have hard surface floors, sweep and wet mop them at least twice a week.

6) The filters of air conditioner/heating systems should be changed or cleaned regularly. A good schedule to follow is once a month during the cold months and twice a month during hot months. If you live in a rental home, and the landlord is responsible for the cleaning or changing schedule, explain to him that your child has asthma and that regular maintenance is essential.

7) Keep the surface dust under control. Dust with a damp cloth weekly. Avoid feather dusters; they don't remove dust; they just stir it up! The new static dusting cloths are quite effective and are disposable. Avoid aerosolized dusting agents. Remember to dust your blinds, silk plants, and lampshades, too.

8) Televisions, computers, and other electronic equipment are dust magnets! Don't forget to clean them when dusting.

9) Curtains can trap a lot of dust. If possible, wash them monthly. If this is not possible because of the type of fabric, at least put them in the dryer for 30 minutes to an hour. This is a very effective way to remove dust.

If you have hard surface floors, sweep and wet mop them at least twice a week.

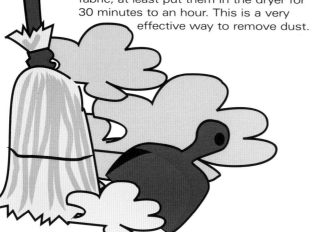

TOBACCO SMOKE

Tobacco smoke is an irritant that should be avoided by anyone with asthma. There have been many studies that indicate that smoking or exposure to secondhand smoke can cause asthma attacks. If you or someone living in your home smokes, the best thing to do is to stop smoking! We understand that this is an incredibly difficult thing to do, and if you or someone living with you can't stop smoking, you should only smoke outside, and never around your child that has asthma! Your child may be exposed to smoke away from home. If you have a babysitter, friends, or relatives that smoke, your child is still being exposed! If any of these people smoke, explain to them that it could trigger an asthma attack in your child, and ask them to cease smoking in your child's presence.

OUTDOOR POLLUTANTS

Air pollution is an outdoor irritant that can trigger an asthma attack. In big cities, especially in the summer months, air pollution levels can be very high. When air pollution in your city or town is high, you need to keep your child indoors as much as possible. This is not a good time for outdoor play or exercise. Other outdoor pollutants include exhaust fumes, campfires, and barbecue smoke. We are not suggesting that you keep your asthma child inside at all times. All children need fresh air and outdoor play! We are trying to make you aware of possible irritants so that you can minimize your child's exposure.

When planning a vacation and choosing a location, be sure to check pollen and air pollution levels!

INDOOR POLLUTANTS

Indoor allergens or irritants are everywhere in our homes. This section should be helpful in recognizing potential triggers and how to remove them or replace them with things that still work; but, are less likely to trigger an asthma attack. Much like air pollution outside, there are things in your home that are pollutants and may be triggering your child's asthma. For many children with asthma, anything with a strong smell may be a trigger. Some of the things that might be bothering your child include: perfume, pine cleaner or bleach, air fresheners, hairspray, scented candles, potpourri, carpet fresheners, incense, and even laundry detergents and fabric softeners. It is best to omit these types of products from your home. When choosing cleaning products, try to find some that are unscented or have neutral smells. Diluted bleach and ammonia are very effective cleansers. Club soda and baking soda work well to remove stains in carpets, upholstery, and clothing. These basic types of cleaning agents are very effective and less expensive than most other products.

Laundry is a big issue for people with asthma. We already addressed the issue of washing bedding, blankets, and stuffed toys in HOT water. We also know that we like our clothes to smell clean and feel soft. However, it is best to use unscented laundry detergent and omit fabric softeners in your laundry routine. If you just can't bear to give up these types of products, at least wash your child's clothes separately in an unscented or hypoallergenic detergent. Do not use fabric softener or dryer sheets. For those of you who work in industry where clothing is saturated with chemicals or strong odors, wash these clothes separately from your child's. If possible, do not line dry bedding. Linens that are line dried pick up outdoor allergens.

Although aromatherapy, scented candles, incense, and potpourri are now considered staples of home decorating, they can be very irritating to your child. To achieve the same ambience that these items provide, try unscented, decorative candles, and limit your aromatherapy to your private bedroom and bath whenever possible.

Air fresheners, ranging from sprays to solids to outlet activated devices, emit strong odors and need to be avoided. Carpet freshener powders, vacuum cleaner fresheners, and air conditioning fresheners should not be used. Baking soda is a good substitute for carpet and vacuum cleaner fresheners. Air conditioner fresheners are particularly hazardous because they can permeate all areas of your home through the ducts. We all strive to have fragrant homes; however, your child's health will benefit from these changes.

> *Much like air pollution outside, there are things in your home that are pollutants and may be triggering your child's asthma. For many children with asthma, anything with a strong smell may be a trigger.*

It is best to use unscented laundry detergent and omit fabric softeners in your laundry routine.

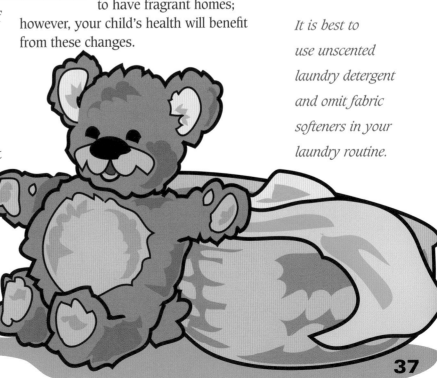

Decreasing indoor irritants is a big challenge for everyone. We all take for granted that items we use on a regular basis are safe and won't lead to health problems. For most people they are. However, on behalf of your child with asthma, you need to begin to think in terms of what household products you use that may be triggering your child's asthma. Like dieters reading food labels, you should be challenged to investigate products as potential triggers and make informed choices. An example would be choosing pump-style hairspray over aerosolized spray, or roll-on deodorant versus spray deodorant.

After taking an inventory of your home and minimizing potential indoor irritants, you need to recognize that your child will still be exposed to these triggers in places other than home. You still have some control by keeping your child away from places that may trigger an attack. This might include hair salons, cleaning product aisles in grocery stores, fabric stores, gift shops that specialize in aromatherapy or scented candles, or perfume counters in department stores. It is different with each child. It all comes down to investigating and zeroing in on what irritants cause your child problems. Once you've identified these indoor irritants, you can go a long way to minimize your child's exposures.

Choose pump-style hairspray over aerosolized spray or roll-on deodorant versus spray deodorant.

INDOOR FUNGI (MOLDS)

Indoor molds are often found in homes that have water leaks or damp and moldy rooms, such as basements. If your child is sensitive to molds, or if you notice that his nose runs, his eyes water, or he starts coughing, wheezing, feeling short of breath, or experiences a tight feeling in his chest when he is in a damp or moldy room, you need to take action. Fix all water leaks, eliminate any water source associated with mold growth, and thoroughly clean all moldy surfaces. Attempt to reduce humidity to fifty percent or less inside your home. Never use a room humidifier or vaporizer in your child's room. Evaporative (swamp) coolers can be harmful to people who are sensitive to both dust mites and/or mold. Because humidifiers, vaporizers, and evaporative coolers increase humidity levels, they encourage the growth of both dust mites and mold.

COCKROACHES

It is a known fact that increased exposure to cockroaches can be an asthma trigger, particularly for inner-city children who may have cockroaches in their bedrooms. It is important to keep your home cockroach-free. Some steps to accomplish this are to never leave food or garbage exposed. Do not let your child eat or keep any type of food or flavored beverage in his bedroom. The best treatment method to rid your home of cockroaches is placing boric acid powder behind your refrigerator, stove, and other areas that your child and pets can't reach. Poison baits and roach traps are also very effective. These types of treatment are better than chemical agents because the chemicals may actually be an irritant for your child. If you must have your home treated chemically, keep your child away from the house during treatment and do not let him return until the chemical odor is completely gone.

OUTDOOR ALLERGENS

If your child has a known allergy to trees, grasses, weeds, or mold, as determined by allergy testing, you will want to reduce his exposure during the time that his allergen sensitivity is the highest. Although this is sometimes unrealistic for children, it helps to stay indoors, with the windows shut and air conditioners on. If your child must be outside, it is better to play or exercise in the mornings or evenings. Pollen and mold counts are typically higher throughout the afternoon. Some children are given medicines, such as anti-histamines and/or decongestants to help with outdoor allergies. If your child has a known outdoor allergen, speak with your doctor about medicines that may help during times of the year when his allergens are at their peak.

Most local news stations and newspapers now give daily reports of the allergen levels. Keep an eye on the levels that your child is sensitive to and limit his outdoor exposure during the times when the allergen is moderate to heavy.

Air conditioning during warm weather is recommended for patients with asthma, because closed doors and windows keep outdoor allergens outside. Central air conditioning also helps control humidity and reduce the growth of house dust mites.

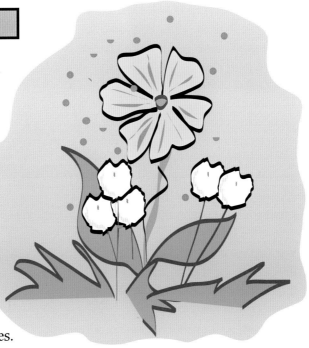

If your child must be outside, it is better to play or exercise in the mornings or evenings. Pollen and mold counts are typically higher throughout the afternoon.

OTHER FACTORS

We have covered a lot of different indoor and outdoor irritants that can trigger your child's asthma. In addition to these environmental triggers, other factors may increase your child's symptoms and the frequency of his attacks:

RUNNY NOSE AND SINUS PROBLEMS A lot of children with asthma have runny or stopped-up noses, or sinus drainage. These upper respiratory problems can cause increased asthma symptoms and eventually asthma attacks. If your child has a chronic sinus problem, you should speak with your child's doctor about using a nasal corticosteroid spray. Some brands include: Nasonex, Flonase, and Rhinocort. They decrease nasal swelling, drainage, and congestion. Your doctor also needs to evaluate your child if he has a sinus problem. Chronic sinus problems sometimes mean that there is an infection and your child may need to be treated with antibiotics. Only your child's doctor can determine if he has an infection. If you suspect this is the case, you need to take him for a doctor visit.

GASTROESOPHAGEAL REFLUX

Gastroesophageal reflux is a condition in which swallowed food or liquid comes back up into your child's esophagus, the food tube that connects the mouth to the stomach. This disorder can lead to asthma symptoms, particularly at night when your child is sleeping. Babies with this disorder will have frequent vomiting. Children and adults may complain of food coming back up their throat and leaving a bile taste in their mouth. If your child has these types of symptoms, you need to tell your doctor. There are different types of medicines used to treat this problem. If your child definitely has this problem, you need to:

Be aware of the dangers associated with taking aspirin.

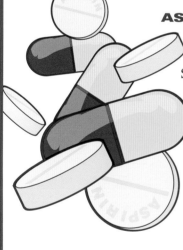

- Keep your child from eating or drinking two to three hours before going to sleep at night.
- Elevate the head of the bed six to eight inches with blocks, or use a wedge type pillow to sleep on.

ASPIRIN SENSITIVITY
It is a good idea to never give aspirin to children. Not only is it linked with Reye's Syndrome, aspirin can cause asthma attacks. A better choice for pain or fever relief is acetaminophen. As children with asthma become adults, they need to be aware of the dangers associated with taking aspirin. If they are sensitive to aspirin, taking it can cause a severe and sometimes fatal asthma attack.

Many patients with asthma are sensitive to foods that contain sulfites.

SULFITE SENSITIVITY
Many patients with asthma are sensitive to foods that contain sulfites, a common preservative in foods and beverages. They can also result in foods that have been barbecued. The most common foods that contain sulfites are shrimp, dried fruit, instant potatoes, processed meat such as hot dogs and bologna, and Chinese food with MSG. If your child shows increased asthma symptoms or complains of a sore throat after eating these foods, he should avoid them. Any child with severe persistent asthma should never eat foods containing sulfites.

BETA-BLOCKERS
Medicines that contain beta-blockers should not be used by asthma patients. Beta-blockers are usually found in heart medicines, but may also be found in some eye drops or ointments. If you have any questions about these types of drugs, do not hesitate to speak to your child's doctor.

INFECTIONS
Viral infections that are associated with flu and colds are the number one triggers for asthma attacks in infants and small children. If your child gets a respiratory infection, you need to have him seen by his doctor. A good way to decrease the incidence of cold and flu is to teach your child to wash his hands thoroughly and frequently with an antibacterial soap. Encourage him to keep toys and other items out of his mouth. Minimize his exposure to other children or adults that are sick whenever possible. Antibiotics do not work against viral infections, but you may want to discuss other modes of therapy with your child's doctor.

WOW! We know this is a lot of information, but we cannot reiterate how important it is to identify your child's asthma triggers and take measures necessary to minimize his exposures. Following these critical steps will help you and your child gain control over his disease and live a healthier life. On the next few pages, Zoey will help your child better understand asthma triggers and things he can do to keep himself symptom-free.

It is hard for me to breathe when . . .

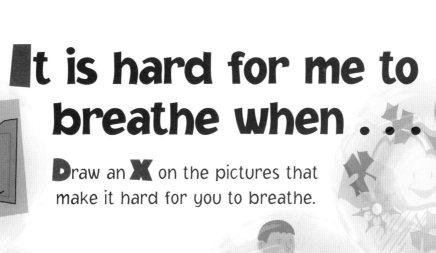

Draw an **X** on the pictures that make it hard for you to breathe.

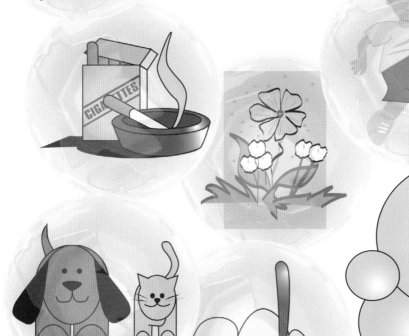

Coughing, wheezing, and shortness of breath are all signs of asthma. Different triggers make your asthma worse. They may even cause an attack. Zoey knows what triggers make it hard for him to breathe, and it is important that you learn your triggers, too.

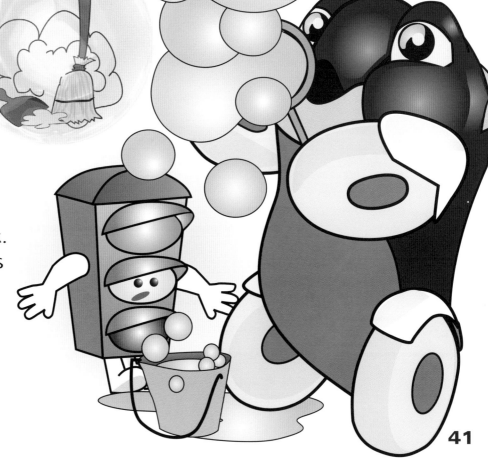

41

Some children are allergic to animals that have
fur, feathers, or hair.

Do you have a pet? ☐ yes ☐ no

Are you allergic to animals? ☐ yes ☐ no

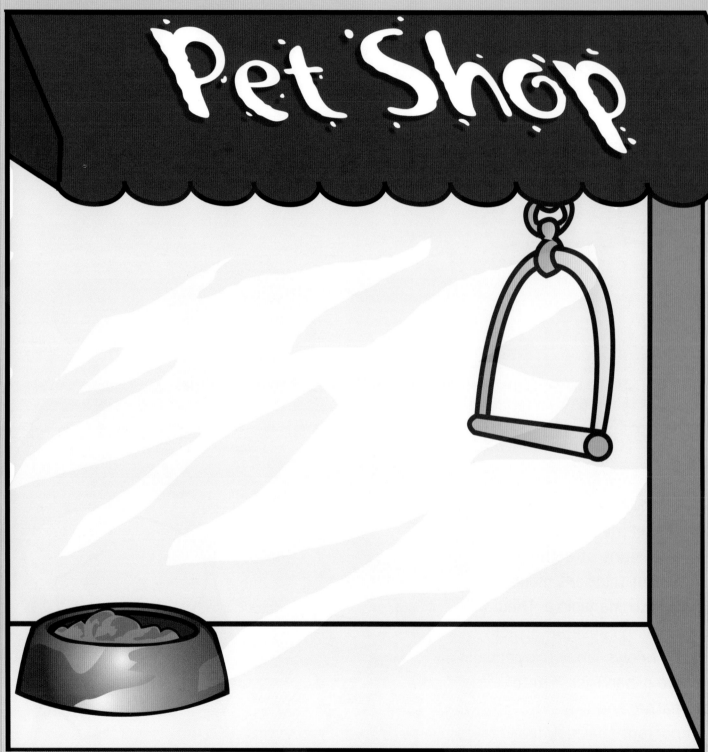

Draw a picture of your pet. If you don't have a pet,
draw a picture of a pet you would like to have.

CHILD'S ACTIVITY

Put an X next to the animals below that have fur, feathers, or hair.

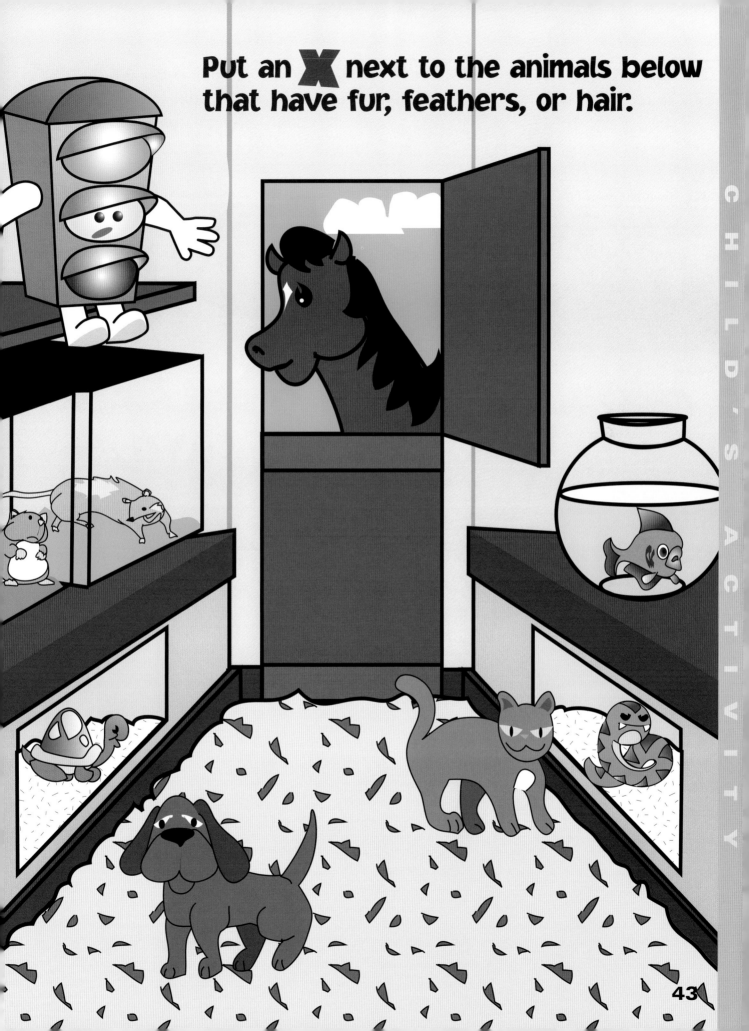

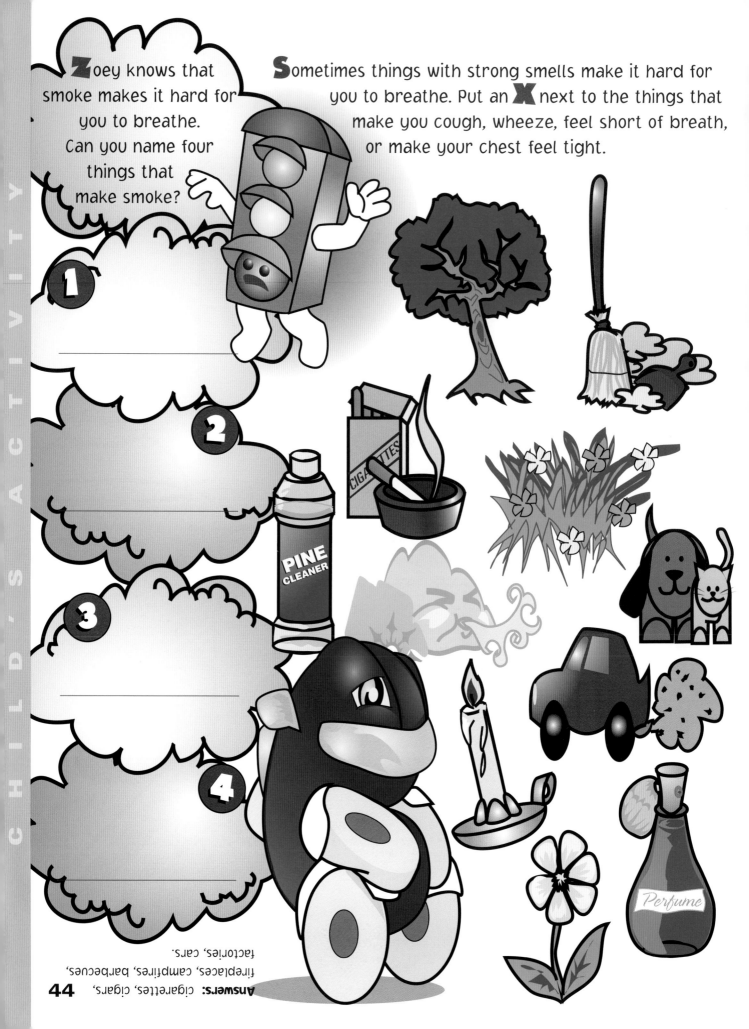

Zoey knows that smoke makes it hard for you to breathe. Can you name four things that make smoke?

1 _____

2

3 _____

4 _____

Sometimes things with strong smells make it hard for you to breathe. Put an **X** next to the things that make you cough, wheeze, feel short of breath, or make your chest feel tight.

PINE CLEANER

CIGARETTES

Perfume

Answers: cigarettes, cigars, fireplaces, campfires, barbecues, factories, cars.

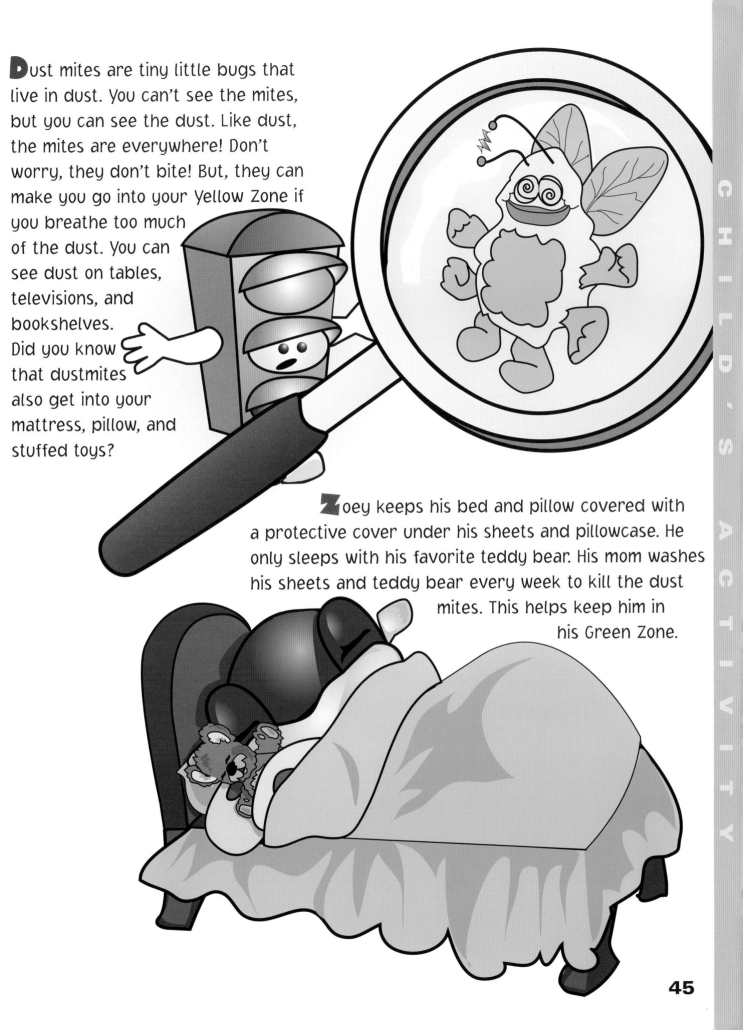

Dust mites are tiny little bugs that live in dust. You can't see the mites, but you can see the dust. Like dust, the mites are everywhere! Don't worry, they don't bite! But, they can make you go into your Yellow Zone if you breathe too much of the dust. You can see dust on tables, televisions, and bookshelves. Did you know that dustmites also get into your mattress, pillow, and stuffed toys?

Zoey keeps his bed and pillow covered with a protective cover under his sheets and pillowcase. He only sleeps with his favorite teddy bear. His mom washes his sheets and teddy bear every week to kill the dust mites. This helps keep him in his Green Zone.

45

Section V Summary

SECTION V - ENVIRONMENTAL TRIGGERS

1. *Environmental triggers are also known as irritants or allergens and may increase asthma symptoms or cause an attack.*

2. *The number one trigger of asthma attacks in babies is upper respiratory infections.*

3. *Home assessments should be performed for anyone that has asthma to minimize potential triggers in their living environment.*

4. *Animals with fur, hair, or feathers have dander that may trigger an attack in some children with asthma. This includes dogs, cats, birds, horses, hamsters, and ferrets.*

5. *Dust mites are microscopic bugs that are everywhere, including bedding, carpets, and upholstered furniture. When breathed in large quantities, they may trigger an asthma attack.*

6. *The pillow and mattress of a child with asthma should always be covered with a protective cover that keeps him from breathing dust mites.*

7. *Tobacco and wood smoke should be avoided by anyone with asthma.*

8. *Air conditioning/heating filters need to be changed every two weeks during warm weather and once per month during cold weather.*

9. *Products with a strong smell, such as carpet fresheners, perfume, pine cleaner, scented candles, and potpourri can trigger an asthma attack.*

10. *Molds are found indoors as well as outdoors. They are typically associated with plumbing leaks, damp basements, or roof leaks. Molds can trigger asthma attacks.*

11. *Room humidifiers or vaporizers should never be used on children with asthma. Humidity levels should be less than 50% in homes at all times.*

NOTES

_____

_____

_____

_____

_____

_____

Exercise

All children need to play and participate in physical activities. For children with asthma, this is often a challenge because their breathing is sometimes affected. There is no formal exercise program designed specifically for children with asthma. Instead, you need to allow and encourage your child to get as much exercise as he can tolerate.

When asthma medicines are used properly, they can be very effective in reducing the occurrence of exercise-induced asthma. For children who experience increased asthma symptoms with exercise, their doctor may prescribe a combination of long-term medicine with rescue medicine like albuterol. We will go into greater detail on these medications and how they are used later in the workbook.

Some parents have a tendency to want to exclude their child from physical activity, because their child has had an asthma attack in the past. There are several pitfalls you may encounter if you regularly exclude your child from play or exercise, including weight gain and low self-esteem, associated with isolation from your child's friends or peers. Obesity causes additional strain on the lungs and puts a child in a cycle of weight gain, difficulty breathing, and inactivity. By not participating in group activities, your child's peers become aware of his illness and begin treating him differently, leading to low self-esteem and stress.

As a parent of a child with asthma, you must remember that all children, even those with chronic illnesses or disabilities, need to live socially active lives. Your job is to work with your child's doctor to create a medicine plan that will allow him to participate in physical activities to the greatest extent possible.

Begin planning activities with your child, keeping in mind the triggers that you have already identified and minimizing his exposures. For example, if your child has sensitivities to tree pollen in the spring, it may not be wise to let him play baseball in the early spring season. Instead, it might be better to let him join a swim club or team that usually practices in an indoor pool. If your child loves soccer but doesn't do well during the hot summer months, consider the fall league versus the spring or summer leagues. Most communities have a host of indoor and outdoor sports activities, available to your child year-round. With some creative planning and community investigation, you will be able to find a physical activity that your child enjoys and which promotes his happiness and health.

Exercise

When you play outside, what are your favorite things to do? Put an X next to your choices.

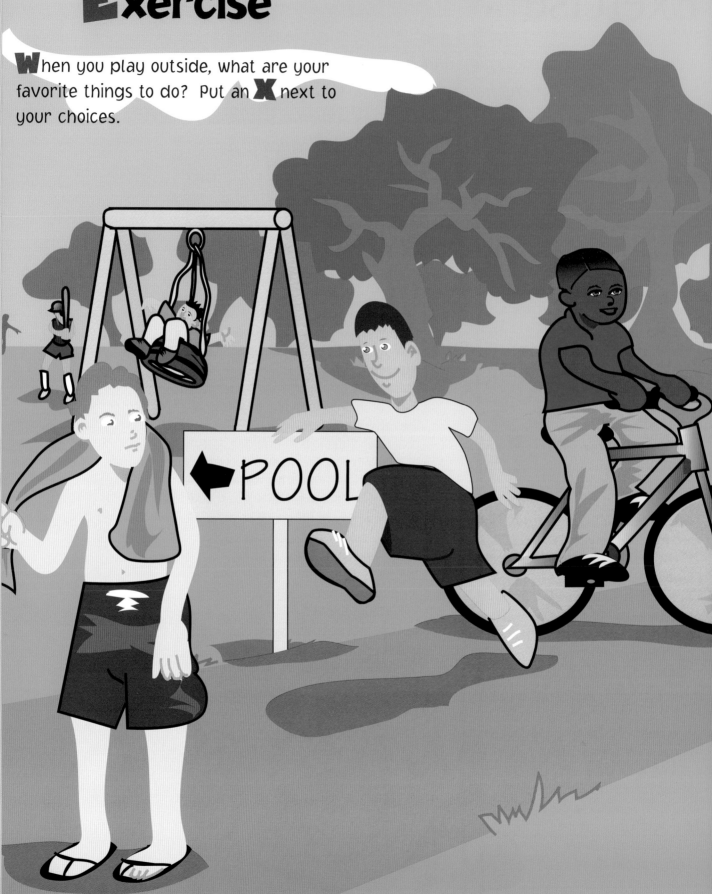

POOL

48

Sometimes, when Zoey is playing, he gets short of breath and starts wheezing! He gets into his Yellow Zone.

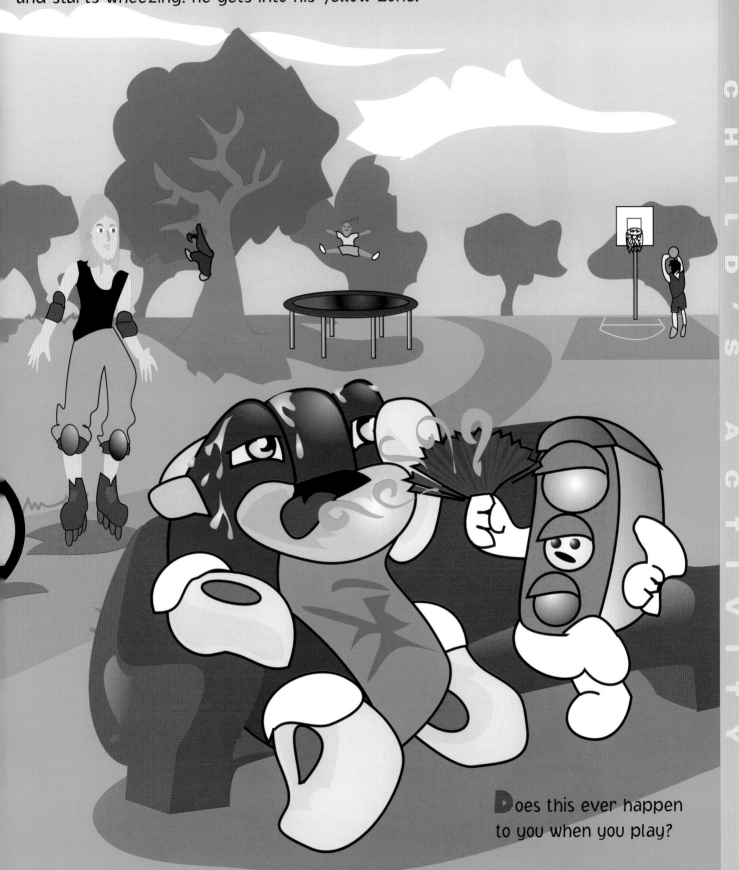

Does this ever happen to you when you play?

49

What sports do you play?

Put an **X** next to your favorite sports.

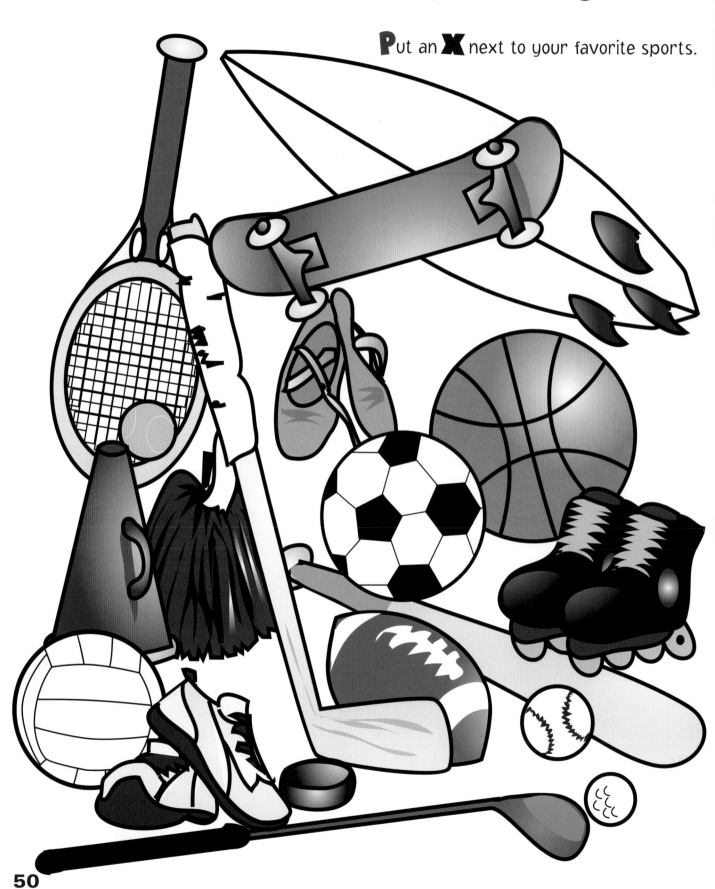

CHILD'S ACTIVITY

Can you remember what makes it hard for you to breathe?

Draw a picture of those things.

Section VI Summary

SECTION VI - EXERCISE

1. Children with asthma should exercise and play.

2. Proper use of asthma medicine may allow your child to participate in exercise, sports, or play without symptoms.

3. It is important to find physical activities that minimize your child's exposure to known triggers.

NOTES

_____

_____

_____

_____

_____

_____

_____

_____

_____

_____

_____

Asthma Medications

One of the most important aspects of managing your child's asthma is compliance with and adherence to your doctor's prescribed medication plan. These medicines will help prevent and control asthma symptoms, decrease the frequency and severity of attacks, and reverse bronchospasm.

There are so many types, brands, and ways to take asthma medicines, that is often overwhelming or confusing to know what to take, when to take it, and how to take it. Our goal is to help you and your child understand the difference between these medicines and how best to use them. Let's begin with the two major types of asthma medications.

The first major category of asthma medications are *Long-Term Control Medications.* They are taken daily on a long-term basis to maintain control of any type of persistent asthma. Earlier in the book, we discussed asthma severity and how important it is for you to know how severe your child's asthma is. If you have determined that your child has a persistent form of asthma, he should be on long-term control medicine. Children with intermittent asthma may never be on this type of medication, or may only use it periodically when they are experiencing an increase in their symptoms. If your child has seasonal allergies that cause asthma attacks, your doctor may prescribe a long-term control medicine during the allergy season.

Long-term control medications, also known as preventative, controller, or maintenance medications, include corticosteroids, non-steroidal anti-inflammatories, long-acting bronchodilators, methylxanthines, and leukotriene modifiers. The very names of these medicines sound like a foreign language! We are not going to spend time teaching the chemical compositions of these medicines. Instead, we want you to learn how to classify which of your child's medicines fall into these categories.

Corticosteroids are the strongest and most effective anti-inflammatory medication currently available.

We start with the *corticosteroids.* This type of medicine comes in metered dose inhalers (MDI's) or nasal sprays. They are the strongest and most effective anti-inflammatory medication currently available. This type of medicine reduces the swelling of airways, a condition that is always present. If prescribed by your child's doctor, this medicine can be one of the most important components in controlling asthma symptoms. Often, patients will stop using this medicine when they feel better. If your child has persistent asthma, do not stop using this medicine. If your child is symptom-free, it is most likely due to the daily use of an inhaled corticosteroid. Never stop using this type of medicine without talking to your child's doctor first.

INHALED CORTICOSTEROIDS

- The most effective long-term control therapy for mild, moderate, and severe asthma
- The risks are minimal compared to their effectiveness
- Reduce side effects by:
  - Using MDI's with a spacer or holding chamber
  - Rinse mouth (rinse and spit) with water after each use
  - Use the lowest dose possible that will control the asthma

Like many drugs, corticosteroids are available in both generic and brand names. Below is a table to help you identify your child's corticosteroid. As drug companies are changing and creating new medicines all the time, there may be additional brand names not listed below.

LONG-TERM CORTICOSTEROID Generic-Chemical Name vs Brand Name
beclomethasone dipropionate
Beclovent MDI Vanceril MDI Qvar MDI Beconase AQ Nasal Spray Vancenase AQ Nasal Spray
budesonide
Pulmicort turbuhaler Pulmicort Respules Rhinocort Nasal MDI
flunisolide
Aerobid MDI Aerobid-M MDI Nasalide Nasal Spray Nasarel Nasal Spray
fluticasone propionate
Flovent MDI or Rotadisk Flonase Nasal Spray
triamcinolone acetonide
Azmacort MDI Nasacort Nasal Spray

Although we will be more concerned about the inhaled corticosteroids and how they are used to control asthma, we want to list the nasal sprays that are often used by children with chronic sinus problems, because many children with asthma have this problem, as well. These children may use both an inhaled corticosteroid and a nasal spray. Your child's doctor will discuss possible side effects of inhaled corticosteroids with you; however, the most common are coughing, hoarseness; and thrush, a yeast infection in the mouth. To prevent your child from getting thrush with their corticosteroid inhaler, he *must* rinse his mouth with water and spit out the water after each use of this medicine.

The second group of long-term control medications is the *non-steroidal anti-inflammatories.* These include cromolyn sodium and nedocromil. Milder than a corticosteroid, they are often prescribed for small children to see if they will adequately control their asthma symptoms. Because of their mildness, it takes anywhere from two to six weeks to see a benefit from their use. In addition, they are often used to prevent asthma symptoms associated with exercise and exposure to known allergens. They are taken through an MDI or nebulizer compressor treatment.

LONG-TERM NON-STEROIDAL ANTI-INFLAMMATORIES Generic-Chemical Name vs Brand Name
cromolyn sodium
Intal MDI or nebulizer solution
nedocromil
Tilade MDI or nebulizer solution

The third group of long-term control medications is the *long-acting bronchodilators.* These medicines are used with anti-inflammatory medicines to control nighttime symptoms of coughing, wheezing, and shortness of breath. They are sometimes used to prevent bronchospasm that may occur with exercise or play. Bronchodilators are medicines that relax the smooth muscle lining of the airways to stop and reverse bronchospasm. This type of bronchodilator has long-acting effects and is *not* used for quick relief in asthma attacks.

LONG-TERM BRONCHODILATORS Generic-Chemical Name vs Brand Name
salmeterol
Serevent MDI or diskhaler
albuterol sustained release
Proventil syrup or tablets Ventolin syrup or tablets
formoterol fumarate
Foradil Aerolizer Inhaler

The fourth group of long-term control medications is the *methylxanthines.* This includes theophylline, which provides mild to moderate bronchodilation in asthma. The sustained release form of theophylline is used almost exclusively for nighttime symptoms. It is most commonly used in conjunction with corticosteroids. Sustained-release theophylline is inexpensive and is sometimes used instead of inhaled corticosteroids as the long-term control medication for asthma. However, this is not the preferred form of therapy. If your child is on theophylline, his doctor must monitor his blood levels of the drug on a regular basis. It is very important that you take your child to his doctor for this testing. Increased levels of theophylline in the blood could result in nausea, vomiting, heart problems, headaches, seizures, and chemical imbalances. It also may cause hyperactivity and sleeplessness.

Theophylline is no longer routinely used because the inhaled corticosteroids are so much more effective at controlling asthma and because monitoring blood levels is required.

The fifth and final group of long-term control medications is the *leukotriene modifiers.* This group of medicine includes relatively new drugs used to treat mild persistent asthma. Singulair is now available in a low dose, chewable tablet for children age two and older. These drugs are considered to be alternative therapy to low-dose inhaled corticosteroids or the non-steroidal anti-inflammatories cromolyn sodium and nedocromil. This group of medicine is classified as anti-inflammatories even though they are not inhaled.

One of the benefits of this medication is that it is taken in a tablet form, not inhaled. Although no specific side effects have been reported, blood tests must be done to monitor liver function for those taking ZyFlo. Your child's doctor must do this testing.

LONG-TERM LEUKOTRIENE MODIFIERS *Generic-Chemical Name* vs Brand Name		
zafirlukast tablets		
	Accolate tablets	
zileuton tablets		
	ZyFlo tablets	
montelukast tablets		
	Singulair tablets	

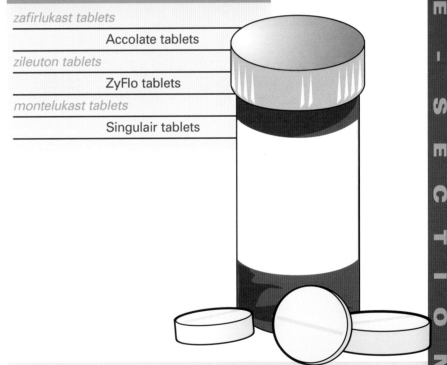

LONG-TERM METHYLXANTHINES *Generic-Chemical Name* vs Brand Name	
theophylline, sustained-release	
	Aerolate tablets
tablets and capsules	
	Quibron-T tablets
	Respbid tablets
	Slo-bid capsules
	Slo-phylline capsules
	T-phyl tablets
	Theo-24 capsules
	Theo-Dur tablets & capsules
	Theo-X tablets
	Theolair tablets & liquid
	Uniphyl tablets
dyphylline	
	Lufyllin tablets, injection, syrup
oxtriphylline	
	Choledyl tablets

LONG-ACTING BRONCHODILATORS

- Salmeterol (Serevent) is very effective at decreasing nighttime symptoms when combined with an inhaled corticosteroid
- Never use salmeterol (Serevent) for an asthma attack or as a rescue medicine
- Proper use of the medicine is critical
- Do not stop using the inhaled corticosteroid with salmeterol (Serevent) even if your child's asthma seems much better

The second major category of asthma medications are the *Quick-Relief or Rescue Medicines*. This category includes the short-acting bronchodilators, anticholinergics, and systemic corticosteroids. The rescue medications are used for quick relief of bronchospasm and the related symptoms, including coughing, wheezing, and chest tightness.

These medications are ***not*** used for long-term control of asthma. Regular, daily use of the short-acting bronchodilators is not usually recommended. If your child is using more than one canister (MDI) of a bronchodilator per month, it is a sign that he might need to start on a long-term control medicine, or increase the use of an inhaled corticosteroid. You should talk with your child's doctor if you think your child falls into this category.

The first group of medicine in the Rescue Medications Category is the *short-acting bronchodilators.* They are the most effective medicines for relieving bronchospasm and preventing asthma attacks that may occur when your child exercises or plays. Like the long-acting bronchodilators, these medicines relieve bronchospasm during an attack by relaxing the smooth muscle that lines the airways. The difference between the two types of bronchodilators is that the short-acting ones relieve bronchospasm typically within thirty minutes, and the long-acting ones take much longer. That is why the short-acting bronchodilators are in the Rescue Medication category and the long-acting bronchodilators are in the Long-Term Control category.

Doctors commonly order this type of medicine for children to use before they exercise, play, or participate in sports or PE. If your child complains of cough, wheezing, or shortness of breath with physical activity, you should ask your child's doctor about bronchodilator therapy with exercise.

Possible side effects with the use of short-acting bronchodilators are increased heart rate, muscle tremors, chemical imbalances, and an increase in stomach upset. Although available in syrup, inhaled forms of this type of medicine, including MDI's and nebulizer solutions, minimize the side effects.

There are many types of short-acting bronchodilators. The most common include:

SHORT -ACTING BRONCHODILATORS *Generic-Chemical Name* vs Brand Name	
albuterol and albuterol sulfate	
	Proventil MDI, nebulizer solution, tablets, and syrup Ventolin MDI, nebulizer solution, tablets and syrup
bitolterol mesylate	
	Tornalate MDI
pirbuterol acetate	
	Maxair MDI
terbutaline and terbutaline sulfate	
	Breathaire MDI Breathine tablets, nebulizer solution, injection Bricanyl tablets and injections
epinephrine	
	Bronchaide Mist over the counter MDI Primatene Mist over the counter MDI
levalbuterol	
	Xopenex nebulizer solution

SHORT-ACTING BRONCHODILATORS

- The most effective rescue medicine for relieving bronchospasm and asthma symptoms
- Increasing use or the use of more than one MDI canister per month shows the need for starting a long-term control medication, or increasing the use of an inhaled corticosteroid
- Regular, daily use of a short-acting bronchodilator is not usually recommended

The second group of rescue medications is the *anticholinergics.* This is medicine commonly known as ipratropium bromide or Atrovent, and is commonly used for patients who have severe asthma attacks. It may also be used as a rescue medication for patients who do not tolerate the short-acting bronchodilators. Side effects of Atrovent may include dry mouth, drying of mucous, and increased wheezing.

The third and final group of rescue medications is the *systemic corticosteroids.* These medicines are used for severe attacks and most frequently in the hospital setting. They are different from the inhaled long-term control corticosteroids discussed earlier in this chapter. These medicines are stronger than the inhaled corticosteroids and are usually taken in tablet or syrup form. They are not taken for long periods of time. Although they are categorized as a rescue medicine, it often takes four hours or longer to see their benefit. Their value in moderate to severe asthma attacks is that they prevent the escalation of symptoms with the attack, speed recovery, and prevent early recurrence of another attack.

There are reversible side effects that may occur with long-term systemic corticosteroid therapy. They typically do not occur with short-term use of these medications. They include increased appetite and weight gain, swelling due to fluid retention, moodiness, increased blood pressure, and stomach ulcers. These side effects generally go away after your child finishes taking the medicine.

RESCUE MEDICATION
SYSTEMIC CORTICOSTEROIDS
Generic-Chemical Name vs Brand Name

methylprednisone

Medrol dose pak tablets

prednisolone

Orapred Oral Solution
Prednisolone tablets
Prelone syrup

prednisone

Deltasone tablets
Prednicin-M 21 pak tablets
Prednisone tablets
Sterapred Unipak tablets

Sometimes your child may be given an inhaler that is a combination of two or more medicines. The most common long-term control combination is the Advair Diskus inhaler. This combines salmeterol and fluticasone. Salmeterol is a long-acting bronchodilator, and fluticasone is a cortico-steroid. However, Advair is typically ordered for children twelve and older.

The most common rescue medicine combination is a Combivent MDI, which includes albuterol and ipratropium bromide. Albuterol is a short-acting broncho-dilator and ipratropium bromide is an anticholinergic.

There are other types of medicines that your child's doctor may order as part of his asthma treatment plan. Nasal corticosteroid sprays are often used to treat chronic sinus problems or runny nose. Anti-histamines and decongestants are often ordered for seasonal allergy sufferers. Although they are not known as asthma medications, when prescribed, they can be an important part of controlling your child's asthma symptoms.

Remember, if your child is being treated with regular prescription medicines, you should always talk to his doctor before giving him any over-the-counter (OTC) medicines.

If your child sees more than one doctor or has been seen in an emergency room or clinic, it is possible that you may have some duplication of medicine. Using the medication charts provided, you will be able to see if your child is on multiple brands of the same type of medicine. If you find this to be the case, you will need to speak to your child's primary doctor for clarification of his medication plan.

This information may seem overwhelming! The first step in understanding and simplifying your child's medication plan is to classify his medicine as "controller" or "rescue." This will be the first activity for your child in this section. He will need your help to do this activity.

Medications

Zoey uses two kinds of
asthma medicine.

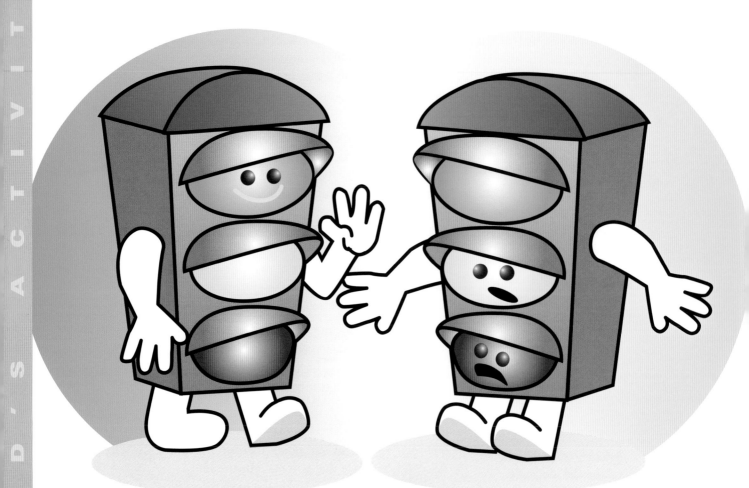

1 **Controllers** - These are the
medicines you take all the
time to keep from having
asthma symptoms or attacks.
Don't stop taking them just
because you feel good! They
keep you in your Green Zone.

2 **Rescue Meds** - These are the
medicines you take only when
you are having an asthma
attack, wheezing, coughing or
feeling short of breath. Take
these when you are in your
Yellow or Red Zones.

Controllers - These medicines keep your airways smooth and wide. They help make the swelling go down.

1. Corticosteroids

- Beclovent
- Vanceril
- Qvar MDI
- Pulmicort
- Aerobid
- Flovent
- Azmacort

2. Non-Steroid Anti-Inflammatories

- Intal
- Tilade

3. Long-Acting Bronchodilators

- Serevent
- Proventil Syrup
- Ventolin Syrup
- Foradil Aerolizer

4. Leukotriene Modifiers

- Accolate
- Singulair

5. Combination Corticosteroid / Long-Acting Bronchodilator

- Advair Diskus

Rescue Meds - These medicines help open the tubes in your lungs when they spasm and get narrow.

1. Short-Acting Bronchodilators

- Albuterol
- Proventil
- Ventolin
- Tornalate
- Breathaire
- Xopenex

2. Anticholinergics

- Atrovent

3. Systemic Corticosteroids

- Medrol
- Orapred
- Prednisolone
- Prelone
- Deltasone
- Prednicin
- Prednisone
- Sterapred

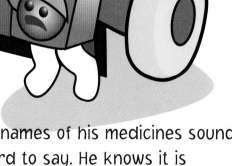

Zoey thinks the names of his medicines sound funny and are hard to say. He knows it is important to learn the difference between his controllers and his rescue meds.

Zoey wants to help you learn which of your asthma medicines are controllers and which ones are rescue meds.

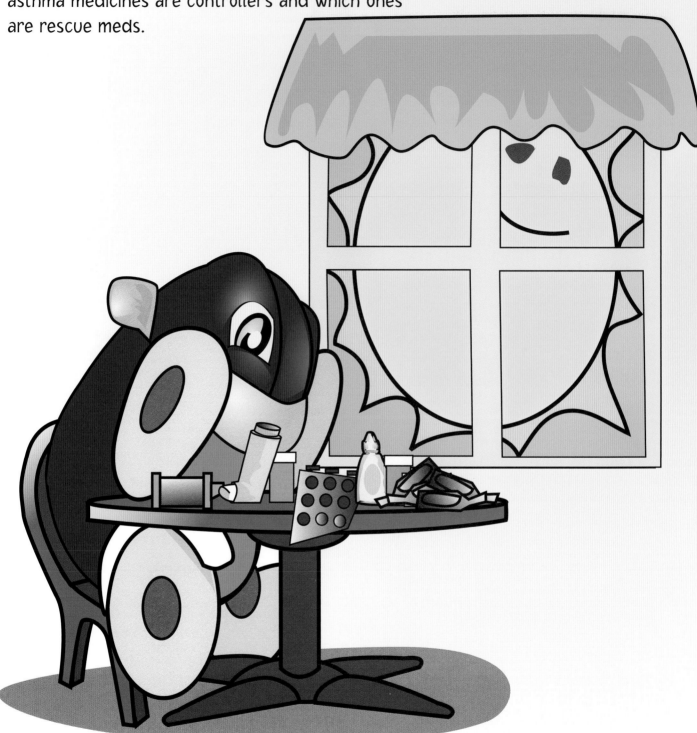

1 Have your Mom or Dad help you do this activity!

2 Get all of your asthma medicines and put them on a table.

3 Look at page 59 to find your medicines. Circle the ones that you take.

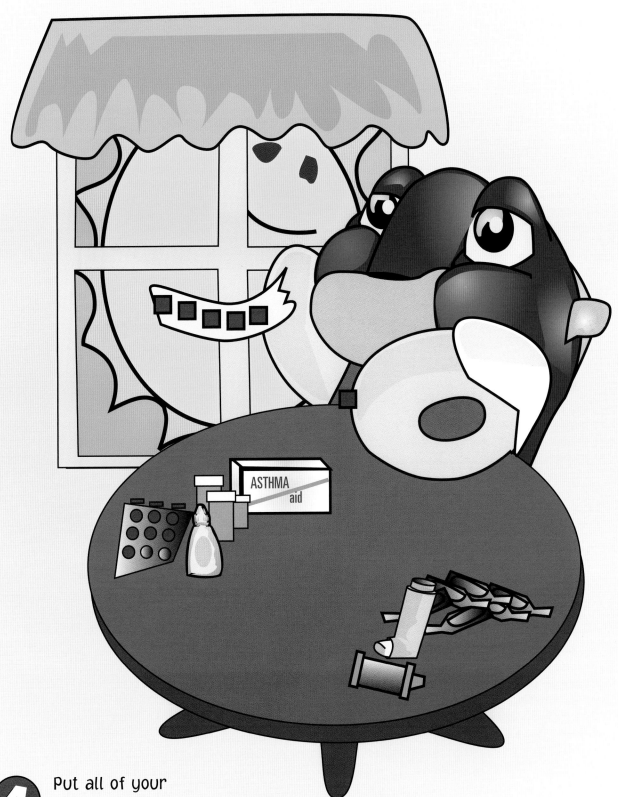

4 Put all of your controllers in one pile and all of your rescue meds in another pile on the table.

Good Job! Now you know which medicines are controllers and which ones are rescue meds. To help you remember, put red stickers on your rescue meds.

61

Fill in the next two charts with your medicines:

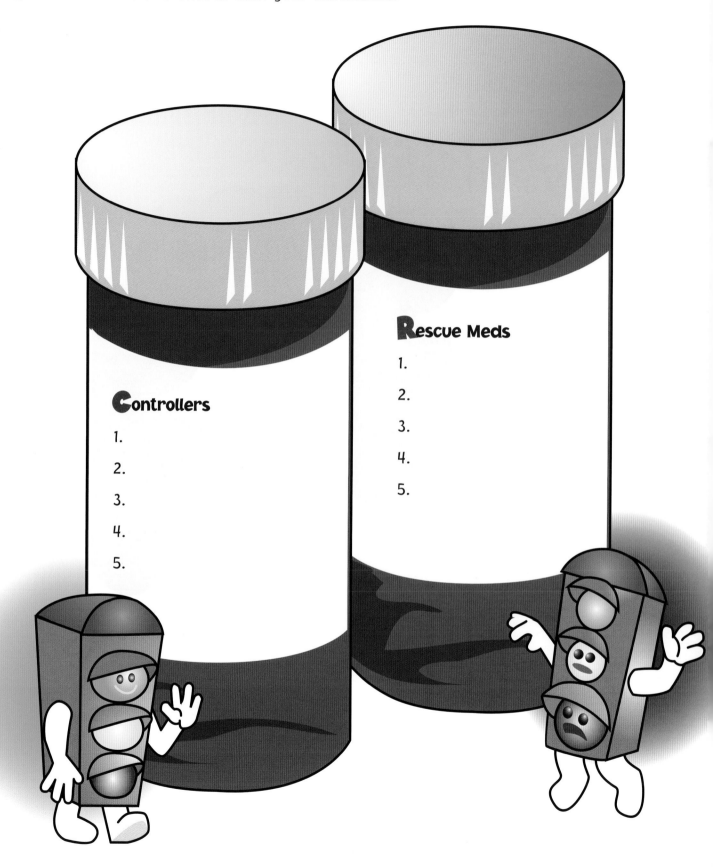

Rescue Meds

1.

2.

3.

4.

5.

Controllers

1.

2.

3.

4.

5.

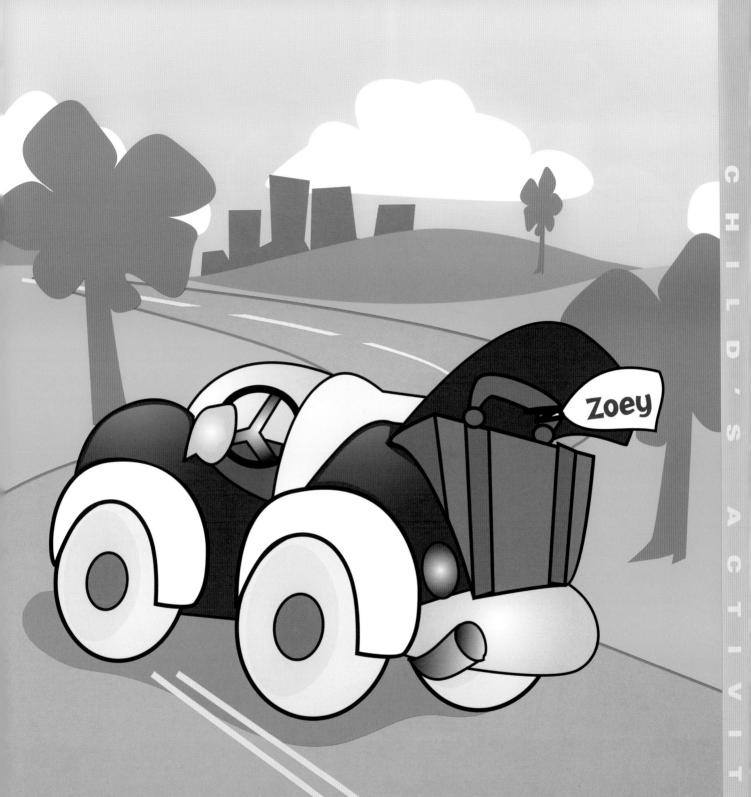

Remember, Controllers are medicines that you take every day. Zoey remembers to take these with him when he goes on vacation, to camp, or on a sleep-over.

63

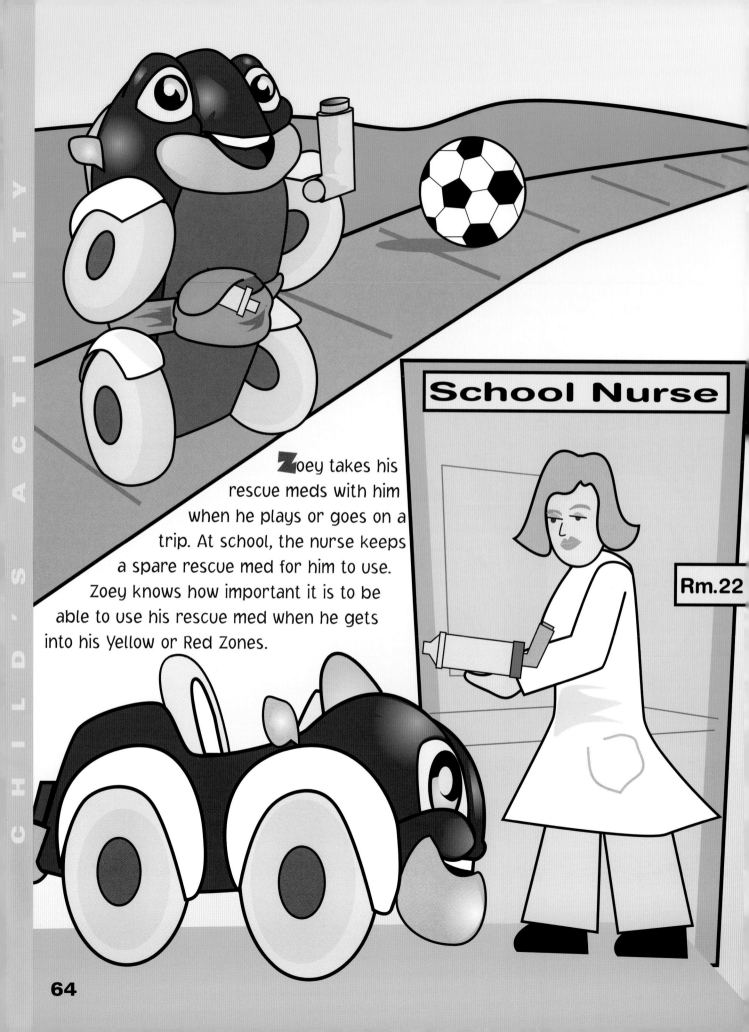

School Nurse

Rm.22

Zoey takes his rescue meds with him when he plays or goes on a trip. At school, the nurse keeps a spare rescue med for him to use. Zoey knows how important it is to be able to use his rescue med when he gets into his Yellow or Red Zones.

Put an **X** next to the things that might make you use your rescue med.

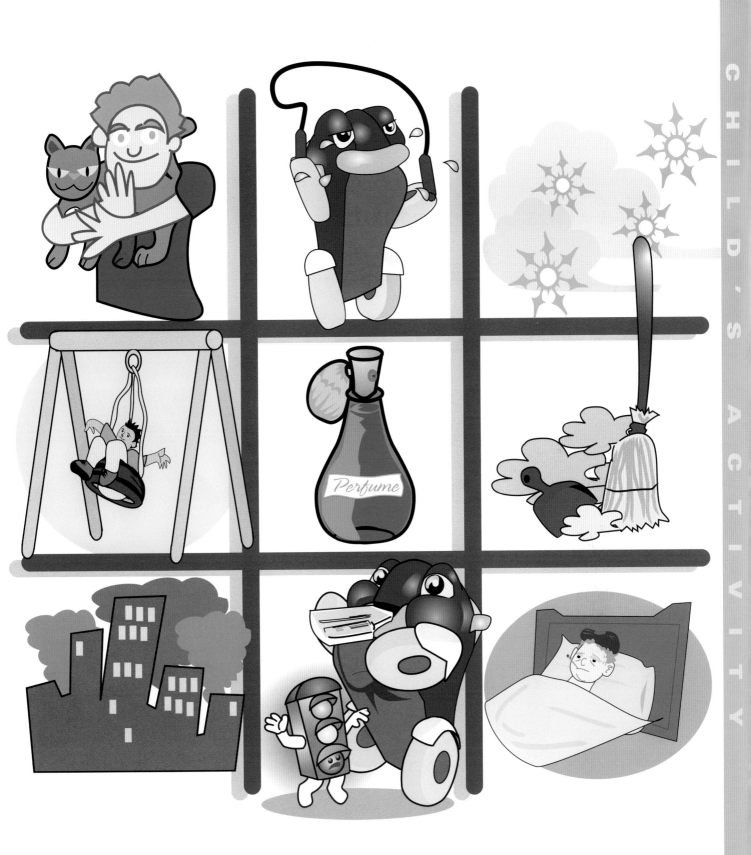

65

Zoey's Secret Message

Instructions: Using the symbol and letter key, can you decode Zoey's secret message?

Code Key

A = 1	n = 14
B = 2	O = 15
C = 3	P = 16
D = 4	Q = 17
E = 5	R = 18
F = 6	S = 19
G = 7	T = 20
H = 8	U = 21
I = 9	V = 22
J = 10	W = 23
K = 11	X = 24
L = 12	Y = 25
M = 13	Z = 26

9   21-19-5   13-25   3-15-14-20-18-15-12-12-5-18

5-22-5-18-25-4-1-25,   5-22-5-14

23-8-5-14   9   6-5-5-12   7-15-15-4.

9   21-19-5   13-25   18-5-19-3-21-5   13-5-4-19

23-8-5-14   9   1-13   23-8-5-5-26-9-14-7,

3-15-21-7-8-9-14-7,   15-18

19-8-15-18-20   15-6   2-18-5-1-20-8.

This is Zoey's secret that keeps him feeling good!

Answer:
I use my controller everyday, even when I feel good.
I use my rescue meds when I am wheezing, coughing, or short of breath.

Section VII Summary

SECTION VII - ASTHMA MEDICATIONS

1. *The two major categories of asthma medications are:*
   - Long-Term Control Medications
   - Rescue Medications

2. *Controller medications are used daily to control asthma, even when your child is feeling good and symptom-free.*

3. *Rescue medications are used during an asthma attack.*

4. *Corticosteroids are the strongest and most effective anti-inflammatory medication currently available.*

5. *Short-acting bronchodilators are the most effective medications for relieving bronchospasm and asthma symptoms.*

6. *If your child uses more than one (1) canister per month of a short-acting bronchodilator, his asthma is not under control.*

NOTES

_____

_____

_____

_____

_____

_____

_____

_____

_____

Medication Delivery Devices

*T*here are different ways to administer the asthma medicines your child takes. Some medicines are in pill or syrup form and do not require any medical device for administration. However, it is important that they be taken as prescribed by your child's doctor. Pay close attention to whether these oral medications should be taken with food or before meals, in the morning or at bedtime.

Asthma medications that are inhaled come in various delivery methods. This includes metered dose inhalers (MDI's), and dry powder inhaler devices. In addition, some inhaled medicines come in a liquid form that are given with a nebulizer compressor treatment.

The most common devices used for inhaled medications are the MDI and nebulizer compressor. They both convert liquid forms of medicine into aerosol mists that your child will inhale into their lungs. We will instruct you and your child on the proper techniques for these devices. If your child uses other devices for inhaled medications, please see your child's doctor, nurse, respiratory therapist, or pharmacist for instruction on the correct use.

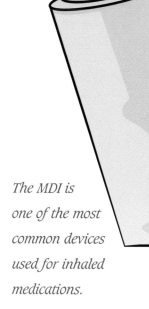

The MDI is one of the most common devices used for inhaled medications.

The preferred method of administration with an MDI includes the use of a "spacer" or a "holding chamber." These devices get their names because they literally provide a space between your child's mouth and the MDI, and hold the medicine until your child takes a breath. For many,

especially children, it is difficult to coordinate the activation of the MDI with taking a deep breath. The spacer makes this procedure easier and more effective by allowing more of the medicine to get into your child's airways and less into the air.

There are many types of spacers available. Some brands that are available include the Respironics Optichamber, Monoghan Aerochamber, and the Inspirease from Key Pharmaceuticals. They are reusable devices that must be ordered or prescribed by your child's doctor. Your child's doctor may have a specific brand that he recommends. Important things to look for are how simple they are to use and how easy they are to keep clean. Do not hesitate to ask the doctor about getting a spacer for your child's use. Many of these devices have either visual or auditory prompts which can motivate your child to use them properly. Some MDI's come with a built-in spacer. When this is the case, an additional spacer is not needed.

One of the greatest challenges with an MDI is knowing when the canister is empty. In the past, the rule of thumb was to drop the canister into a cup of water and if it floated, it was empty. This method is not reliable!

The best way is to date the MDI with the first date it was used. Insert packaging that comes with the MDI will tell you how many puffs are in the canister. You will then need to calculate how long the medicine will last.

For example:

Puffs in Canister = 240

Dose = 4 puffs twice per day

240 / 8 = 30 days

This canister will last approximately 30 days.

This technique works well for medicines used on a regular basis such as your child's inhaled corticosteroids. For medications used on a PRN or "as needed" basis, such as short-acting bronchodilators or other rescue medicine, keeping track is a little more difficult. For these types of inhalers, you may want to purchase a dose counter. Ask your doctor or asthma educator about this handy tool. It is a good idea to always keep a spare rescue inhaler on hand!

You and your child will become very familiar with which MDI is a controller medicine and which one is a rescue medicine. However, other people will not know the difference. We suggest that you mark the rescue MDI with a red sticker. Make sure your child, his school, or daycare provider, and other caregivers including relatives, know that the rescue medicine with the red sticker is the drug to use when your child is experiencing increased symptoms or an asthma attack. In an emergency situation, this can save precious time!

Some asthma patients use nebulizer compressors for inhaled medication treatments. This is a combination of an air compressor (electric or battery operated) and a nebulizer medication circuit. Most insurance companies will purchase one compressor every five years for your child. It is important to find a machine that has a five-year manufacturer warranty. Some of the manufacturers that offer this type of warranty on their compressors include

DeVilbiss (Pulmo-Aide), Respironics (Inspiration) and Medical Industries of America (Sports Neb).

The nebulizer component is a plastic circuit that attaches to the compressor and has a built-in medicine cup. It can be used with a mouthpiece or mask. These circuits are usually disposable and most insurance companies will pay for two circuits per month. With proper cleaning and use, these circuits will last for at least this long, and sometimes longer.

When the compressor is turned on, air moves through the plastic tubing into the medicine cup. The liquid medicine is then aerosolized, and your child breathes it into his lungs through a mouthpiece or a mask. Masks are used for small children who cannot properly use the mouthpiece. Mouthpieces are used when the child is able to hold it upright and seal his lips around it.

Most insurance companies will not purchase a second compressor for use in school or daycare. In addition, the treatment typically takes fifteen to twenty minutes and the school nurse does not have the time to give this type of treatment. Because of the rise in asthma, many schools have numerous children with this disease, yet there is only one nurse. As a result, you need to be sensitive to how much time the school nurse can spend with your child. For this reason, whenever possible, we recommend that you discuss the use of an MDI instead of a nebulizer compressor at the school.

Throughout the next few pages, Zoey will be teaching your child about the proper use of these delivery devices. Zoey will also explain the proper cleaning of these devices. Properly cleaning the spacers and nebulizer circuits is critical in preventing infections. Read through the instructions with your child and have him demonstrate the techniques to make sure he understands how to use his medicines properly. Adherence to your child's prescribed medicine plan is critical to managing his asthma.

Inhalers

How many words can you make from these names?

Inhalers

Metered Dose Inhaler

Spacer

Holding Chamber

1. _____

2. _____

3. _____

4. _____

5. _____

6. _____

7. _____

8. _____

9. _____

10. _____

11. _____

12. _____

13. _____

14. _____

15. _____

16. _____

17. _____

18. _____

19. _____

20. _____

21. _____

22. _____

23. _____

24. _____

25. _____

26. _____

27. _____

28. _____

29. _____

30. _____

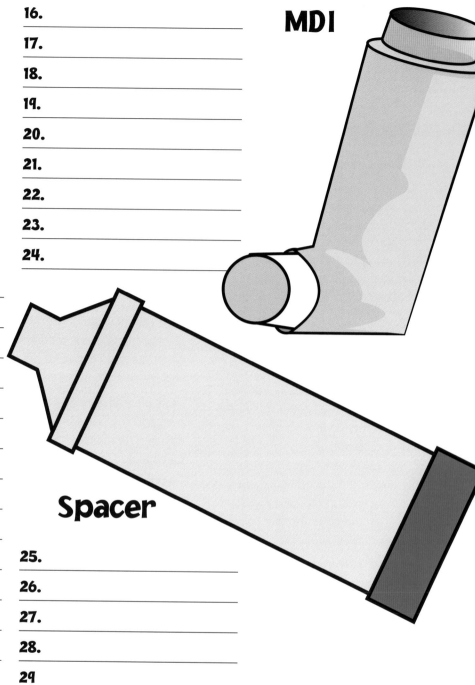

MDI

Spacer

Many of your asthma medicines may be inhalers or metered dose inhalers (MDI's). These are medicines that you breathe into your lungs through your mouth. Zoey always uses a spacer or holding chamber with his inhalers. He will show you how to use your inhalers the right way.

1

Remove the cap of the inhaler and attach the spacer.

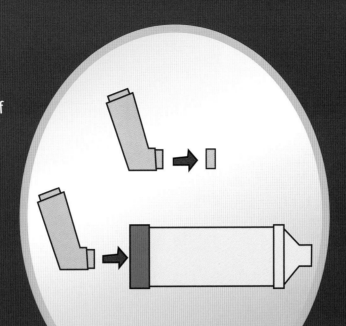

2

Shake the inhaler and spacer at least 4-5 times.

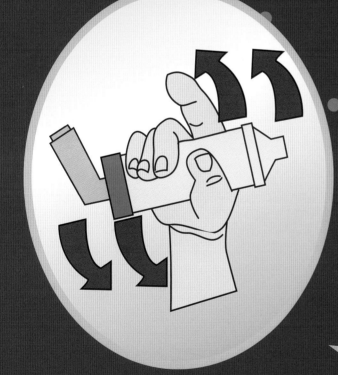

3 Stand up tall

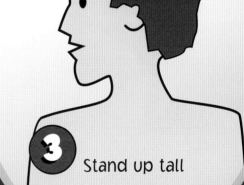

Have a separate spacer for the controller med and one for the rescue med.

4 Exhale slowly to empty your lungs.

5 Put the spacer in your mouth and seal your lips around the mouthpiece. Press down on the inhaler to spray the medicine and breathe in slowly through your mouth, not your nose.

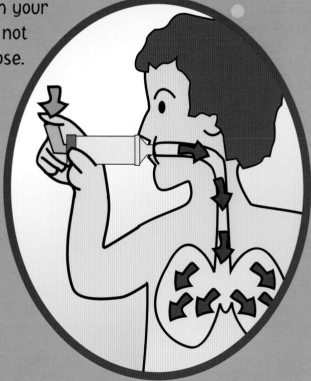

6 Hold your breath and count to 10. This helps the medicine get deeper into your lungs.

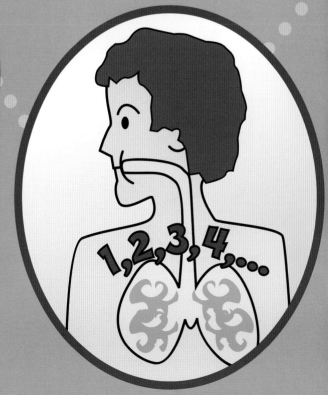

1,2,3,4,....

CHILD'S ACTIVITY

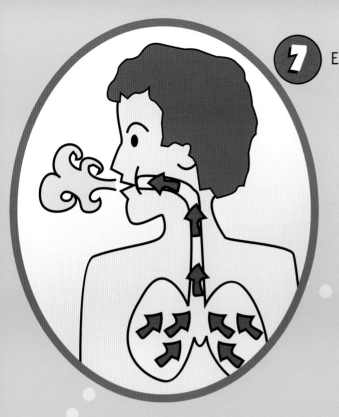

7 Exhale.

8 Wait 1 minute before your next puff.

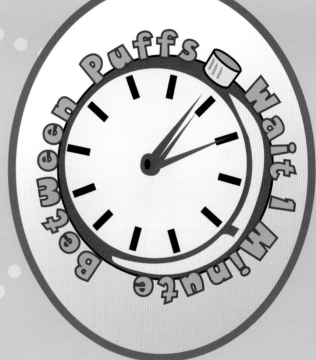

Wait 1 Minute Between Puffs

9 Give yourself the number of puffs your doctor ordered.

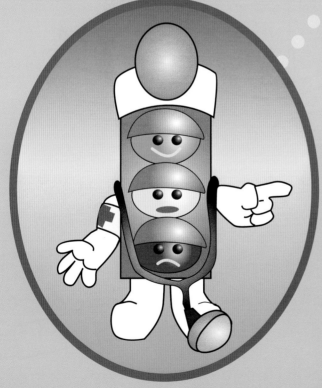

IMPORTANT

After using your corticosteroid inhaler, rinse your mouth with water and spit it out in a sink.

You need to clean your spacer with dish soap and warm water every day. Let it air dry.

IMPORTANT: For complete information, including cautions, refer to the device and medication instructions.

Nebulizers

Connect the dots.

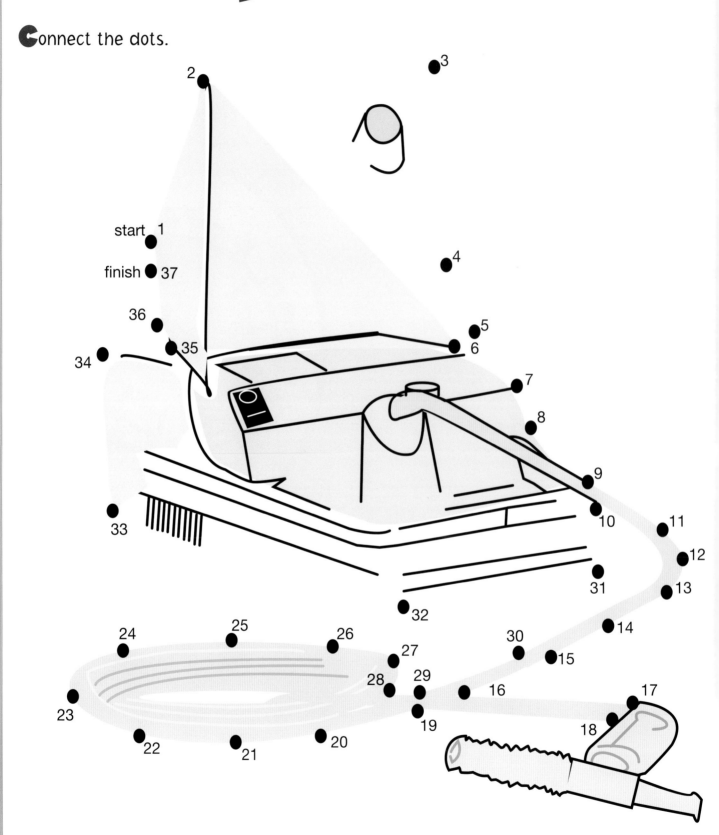

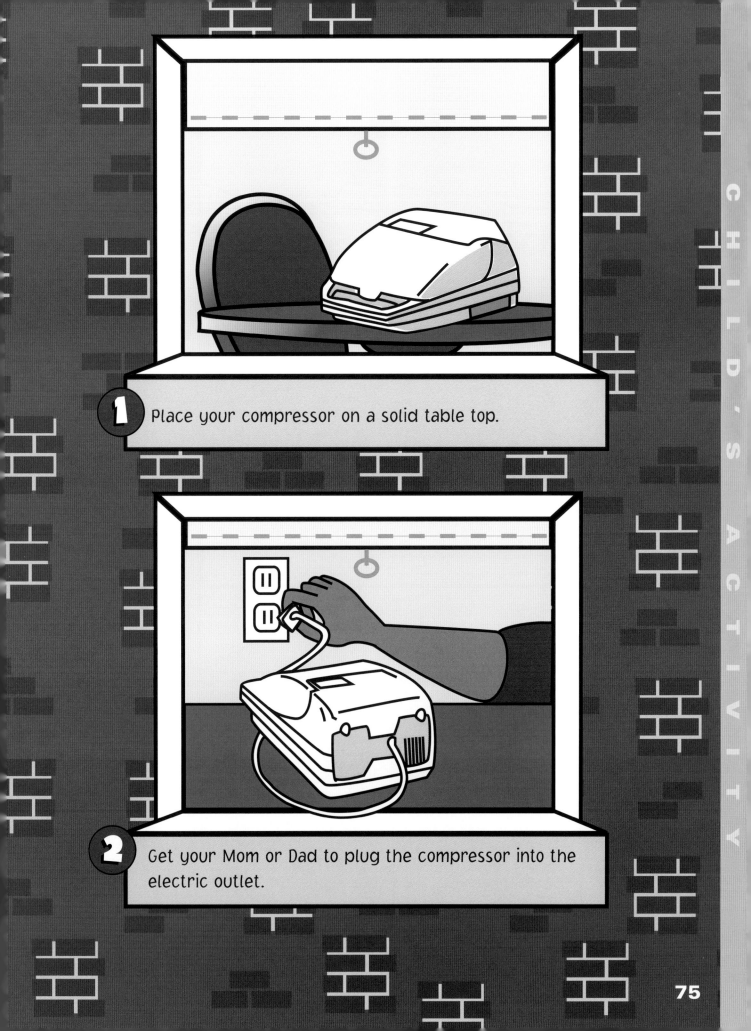

1 Place your compressor on a solid table top.

2 Get your Mom or Dad to plug the compressor into the electric outlet.

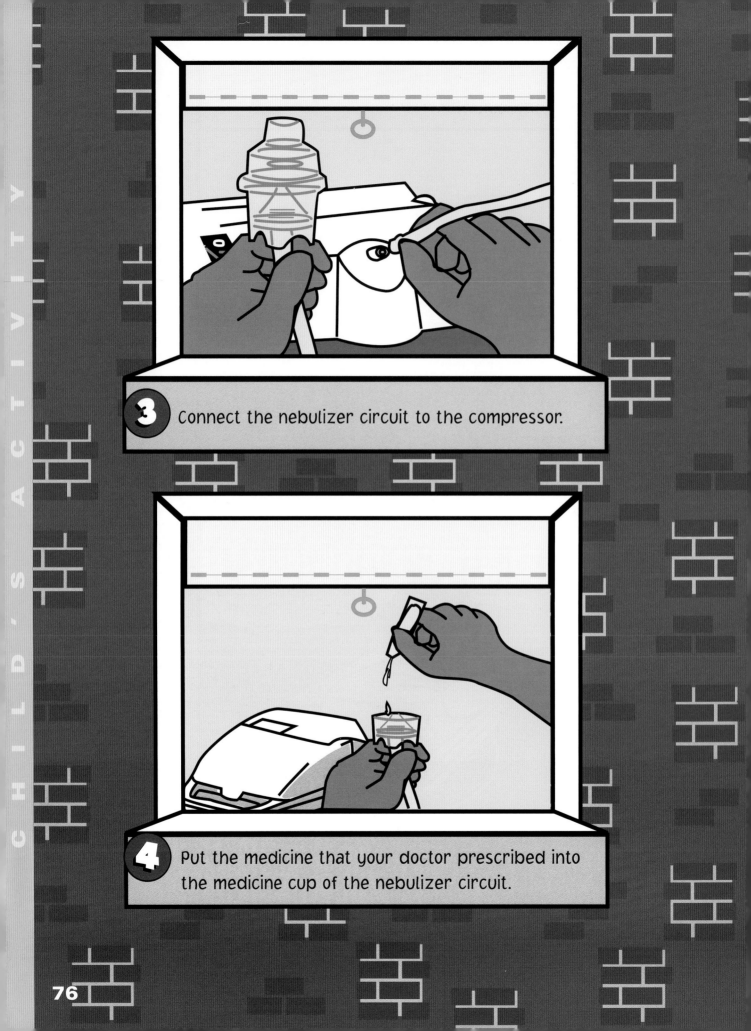

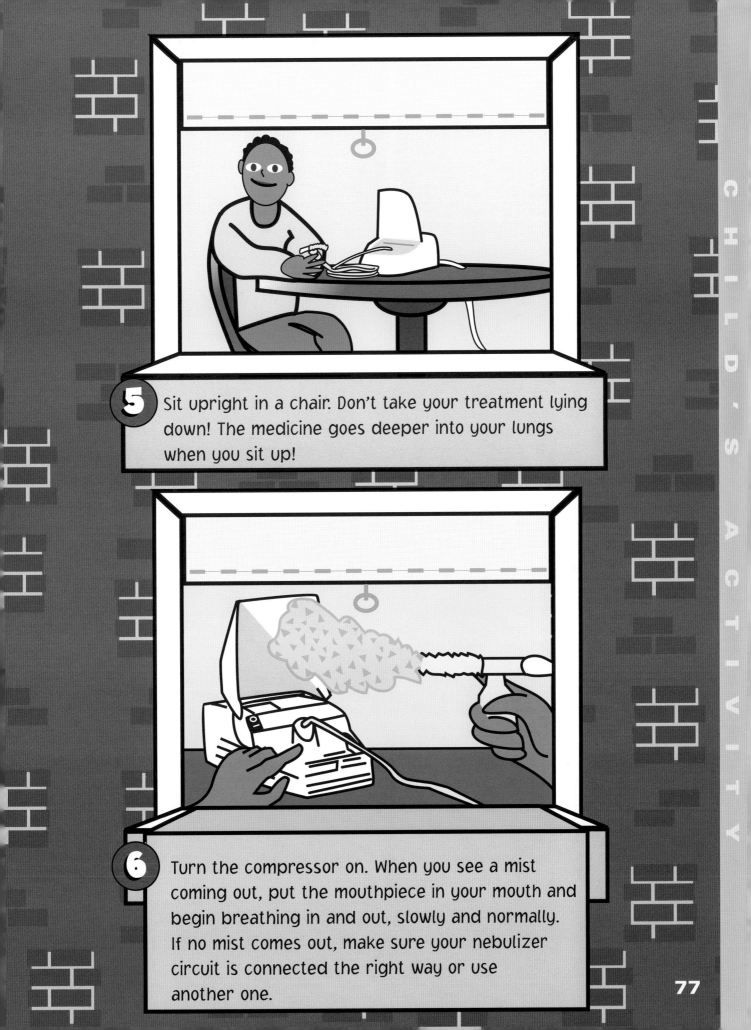

5 Sit upright in a chair. Don't take your treatment lying down! The medicine goes deeper into your lungs when you sit up!

6 Turn the compressor on. When you see a mist coming out, put the mouthpiece in your mouth and begin breathing in and out, slowly and normally. If no mist comes out, make sure your nebulizer circuit is connected the right way or use another one.

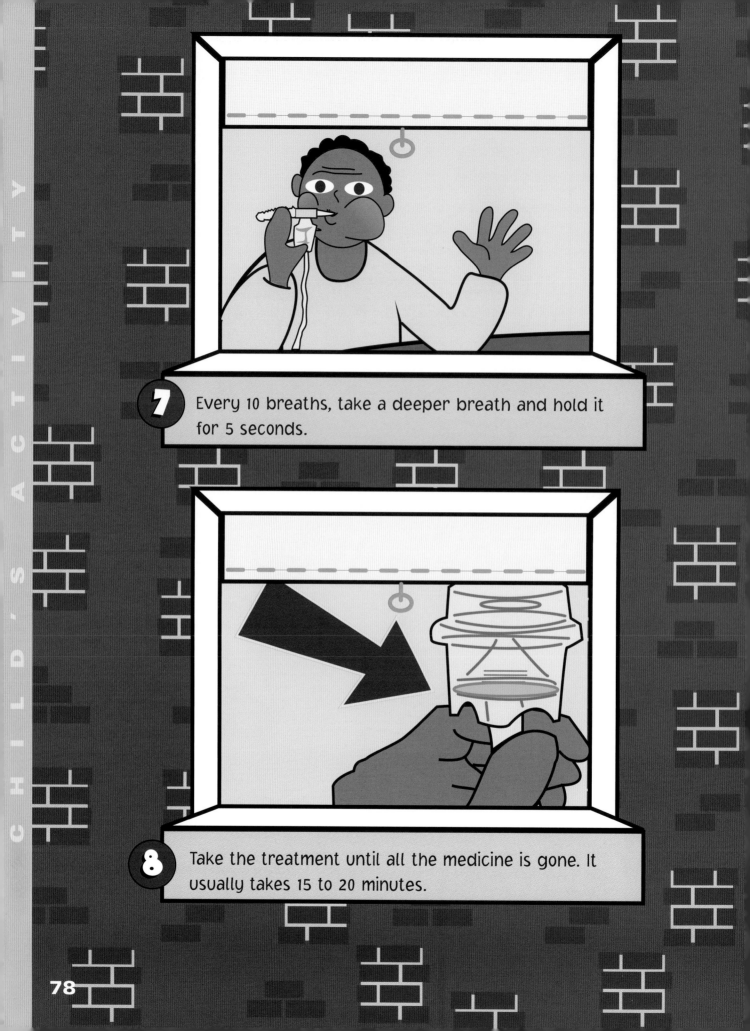

7 Every 10 breaths, take a deeper breath and hold it for 5 seconds.

8 Take the treatment until all the medicine is gone. It usually takes 15 to 20 minutes.

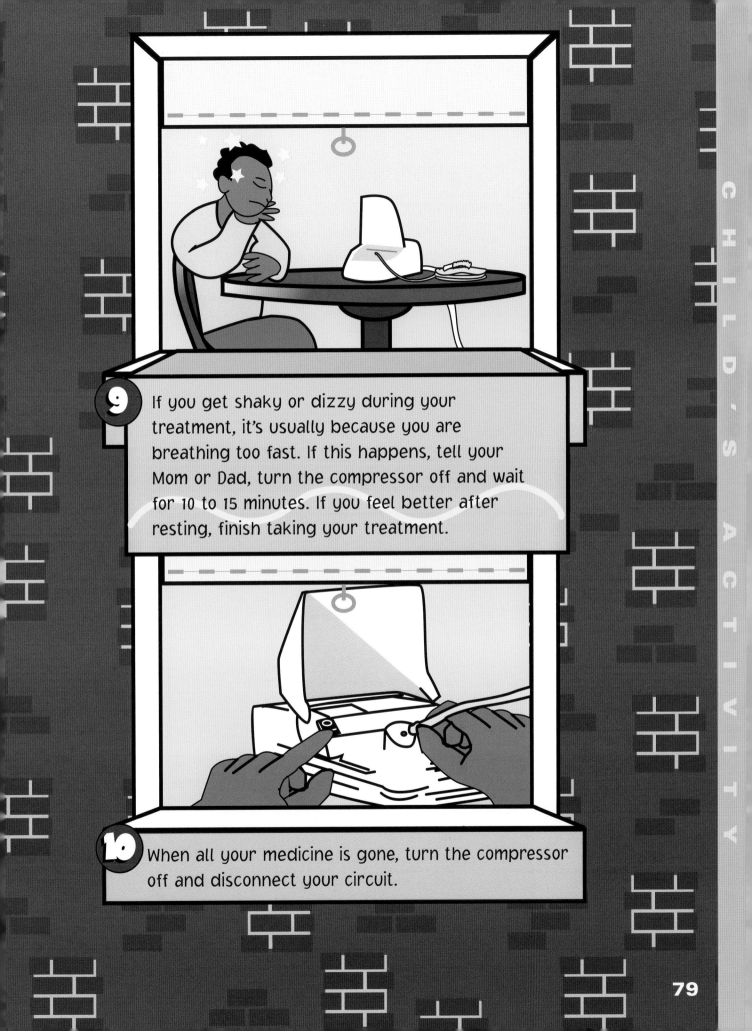

9 If you get shaky or dizzy during your treatment, it's usually because you are breathing too fast. If this happens, tell your Mom or Dad, turn the compressor off and wait for 10 to 15 minutes. If you feel better after resting, finish taking your treatment.

10 When all your medicine is gone, turn the compressor off and disconnect your circuit.

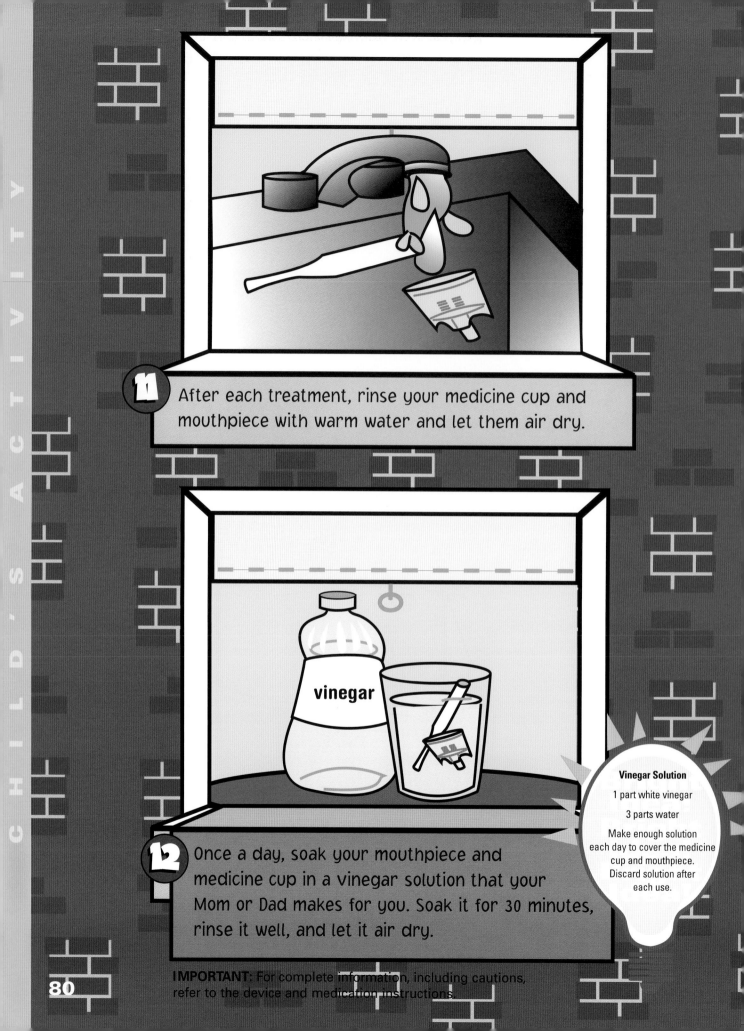

11 After each treatment, rinse your medicine cup and mouthpiece with warm water and let them air dry.

vinegar

12 Once a day, soak your mouthpiece and medicine cup in a vinegar solution that your Mom or Dad makes for you. Soak it for 30 minutes, rinse it well, and let it air dry.

Vinegar Solution

1 part white vinegar

3 parts water

Make enough solution each day to cover the medicine cup and mouthpiece. Discard solution after each use.

IMPORTANT: For complete information, including cautions, refer to the device and medication instructions.

Section VIII Summary

SECTION VIII - MEDICATION DELIVERY DEVICES

1. The nine steps for the correct use of an MDI with spacer include:
- Remove the cap of the inhaler and attach it to the spacer.
- Shake the inhaler 3-5 seconds.
- Stand up tall.
- Exhale slowly until your lungs are empty.
- Put the spacer in your mouth and seal it with your lips. Press down on the inhaler to release the medicine into the spacer and breathe in slowly through your mouth, not your nose.
- Hold your breath and count to 10. This lets the medicine get deeper into your lungs.
- Remove the spacer and MDI from your mouth and exhale.
- Wait 1 minute before your next puff.
- Give yourself the number of puffs your doctor ordered.

2. After using a corticosteroid inhaler, rinse your mouth with water and spit into a sink. Use separate spacers for your corticosteroid and other inhalers.

3. Nebulizer circuits should be cleaned daily with a vinegar solution.

NOTES

_____

_____

_____

_____

_____

_____

_____

_____

_____

Good news! *There are very few foods that trigger asthma. According to the International Food Information Council Foundation, only 6 to 8% of children with asthma have sensitivities to foods that may trigger an attack. Instead of focusing on problem foods, we feel it is important to discuss the merits of a well-balanced, nutritional diet. There is no diet specifically designed for children with asthma.*

A nutritional diet, full of fruits and vegetables, is essential for proper health and weight management. While fats, excess sugar, and "junk" foods need to be limited in all of our diets, children enjoy the taste and fun of these occasional treats. Totally depriving your child of these types of food may potentially lead to a sense of isolation from their friends and peers. Your child's doctor or a dietician can help you plan an appropriate diet for healthy growth and development.

Although very few children have asthma attacks triggered by food, it is important to understand that those with persistent severe asthma or those who experience severe attacks are at risk of an attack when they eat sulfites. Though sulfites are not allergens, they are irritants. They may occur naturally in food or be an additive to foods. The FDA requires a warning label on all foods containing substantial sulfite levels. Read the food labels, especially on dried fruits or vegetables, packaged or prepared potatoes, bottled lemon or lime juice, shrimp, and pickled foods, such as pickles and relishes. In addition to the food preservative sulfites, yellow and red food coloring, and the flavor enhancer, MSG, often used in oriental cooking, may trigger an asthma attack. Besides food, sulfites are found in some medications. As a result, you need to inform your pharmacist that your child has asthma when getting any prescription or over-the-counter drugs for your child.

One final thought on proper diet, you should always encourage your child to drink water. He needs six to eight glasses every day. This not only cleanses the body's systems, but also helps to thin mucous secretions produced in the lungs.

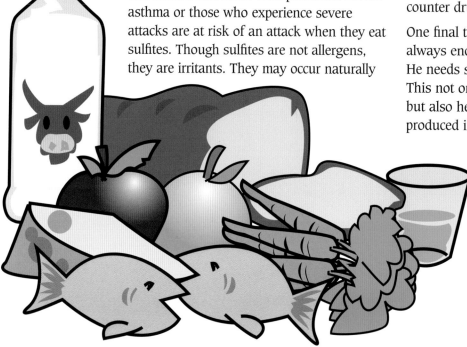

Nutrition

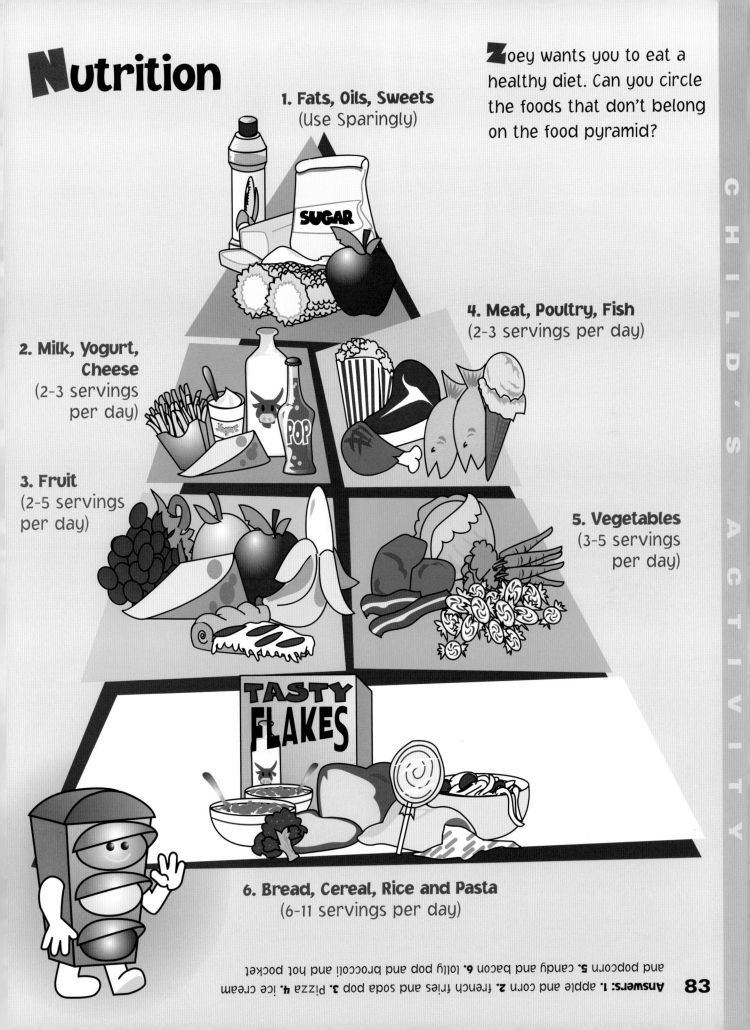

Zoey wants you to eat a healthy diet. Can you circle the foods that don't belong on the food pyramid?

1. Fats, Oils, Sweets
(Use Sparingly)

4. Meat, Poultry, Fish
(2-3 servings per day)

2. Milk, Yogurt, Cheese
(2-3 servings per day)

3. Fruit
(2-5 servings per day)

5. Vegetables
(3-5 servings per day)

6. Bread, Cereal, Rice and Pasta
(6-11 servings per day)

Answers: 1. apple and corn **2.** french fries and soda pop **3.** pizza **4.** ice cream and popcorn **5.** candy and broccoli and hot pocket **6.** lolly pop and bacon

Now that you know what the food groups are and how much of them you should eat, Zoey needs your help finishing this crossword puzzle.

CLUES:

Across

2. I should eat 3 to 5 servings of _____ per day.

5. _____ are fruit that come in a bunch.

7. Too much _____ can give me cavities.

8. _____ makes your bones strong.

Down:

1. My Mom fries food in _____.

3. My Mom scrambles _____ for breakfast.

4. I should drink 6 to 8 glasses of _____ each day.

6. I shouldn't eat a lot of _____ food.

84

C H I L D ' S   A C T I V I T Y

Section IX Summary

SECTION IX - NUTRITION

1. *There are very few foods that trigger asthma.*

2. *If your child has a persistent classification of asthma, they should avoid foods that contain sulfites because they can trigger an asthma attack. These foods include:*
   - Packaged or processed potatoes
   - Yellow or red food coloring
   - Shrimp
   - Pickled foods or relishes
   - Foods containing MSG

3. *Children with asthma should drink 8 to 10 glasses of water per day to cleanse the body's systems and thin mucous secretions produced in the lungs.*

NOTES

_____

_____

_____

_____

_____

_____

_____

_____

_____

_____

Stress and Relaxation

Medical researchers are still trying to determine if stress or other psychological factors may cause children to develop asthma. While this area of asthma research is still being investigated, it is much clearer that these factors can cause an attack in those that have already been diagnosed with asthma. As a parent of a child with asthma, you may have witnessed this type of trigger.

Extreme emotion, such as crying or laughing, sometimes makes breathing more difficult in children with asthma. All children cry and laugh, and we certainly don't suggest that you attempt to stop these normal emotional expressions. However, it is important to know that they may cause difficulty in breathing. It is also important to be prepared to react to your child with calming techniques and rescue medications.

In addition to causing an attack, anxiety, fear, and panic can result from an asthma attack. It is very important that you remain calm and level headed whenever your child is experiencing shortness of breath. If you panic, your child's anxiety will increase, making breathing that much more difficult. Your child needs you to reassure and care for him throughout the episode. Staying calm, speaking softly, and acting confidently diminishes the panic aspect of your child's attack.

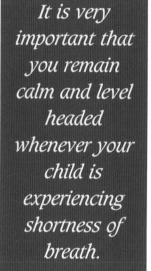

It is very important that you remain calm and level headed whenever your child is experiencing shortness of breath.

Another aspect in stress and anxiety for children with any form of chronic illness is a sense of isolation and being "different" from their friends and peers. These feelings can lead to depression and behavior issues that may result in non-compliance with medications and the overall asthma treatment plan. This is common for children entering puberty. Raising any adolescent is a challenge. Those with chronic illnesses present a separate host of problems. These children often rebel against their disease by not taking their medicines, ignoring symptoms, and exposing themselves to known triggers.

In young children, feelings of depression or defiant behavior usually result from a change in lifestyle that may include a decreased ability to play; restriction from pets, stuffed toys, favorite blankets, or pillows; and the adherence to a regular medication program.

No matter your child's age, it is important to recognize signs of stress, anxiety, and depression so that you can take action to resolve these issues. If you feel overwhelmed or unsure about your child's behavior, or if his health is deteriorating, seek help from your child's doctor, counselor, or clergy. Because stress and anxiety can negatively impact your child's health, it is always important to discuss your concerns with your child's doctor.

In the next few pages, Zoey will be teaching you and your child some techniques for lessening the fear and panic that often occurs with shortness of breath.

Consider calling or making an appointment to visit your child's doctor alone to discuss emotional or behavioral issues that may be affecting his health.

Stress & Relaxation

When Zoey is having an asthma attack, he feels scared. It is scary when you can't catch your breath. Zoey knows how to do things that keep him calm even when he is short of breath. With practice, you can learn these things, too.

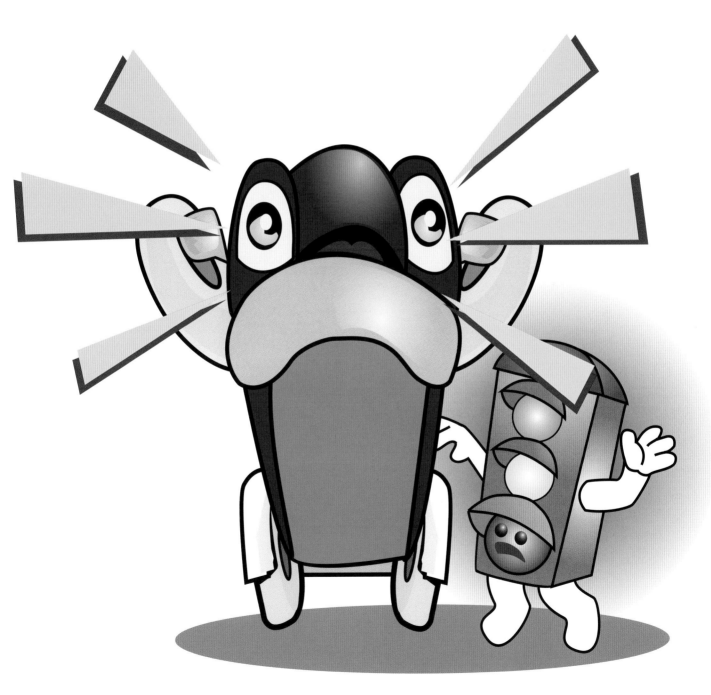

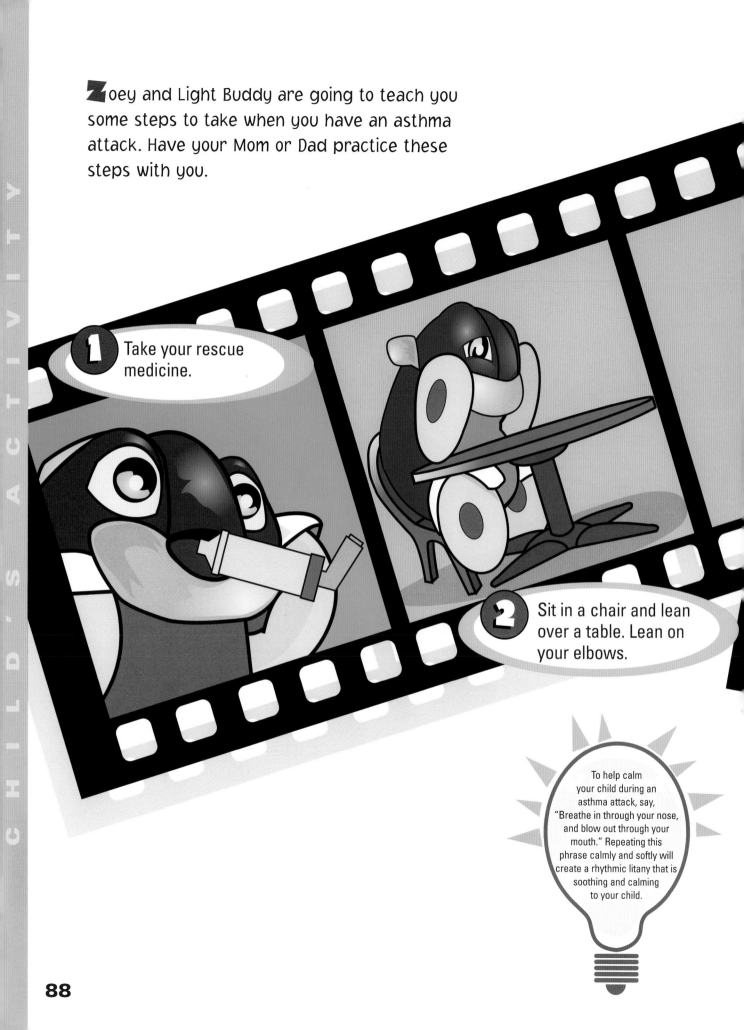

Zoey and Light Buddy are going to teach you some steps to take when you have an asthma attack. Have your Mom or Dad practice these steps with you.

1 Take your rescue medicine.

2 Sit in a chair and lean over a table. Lean on your elbows.

To help calm your child during an asthma attack, say, "Breathe in through your nose, and blow out through your mouth." Repeating this phrase calmly and softly will create a rhythmic litany that is soothing and calming to your child.

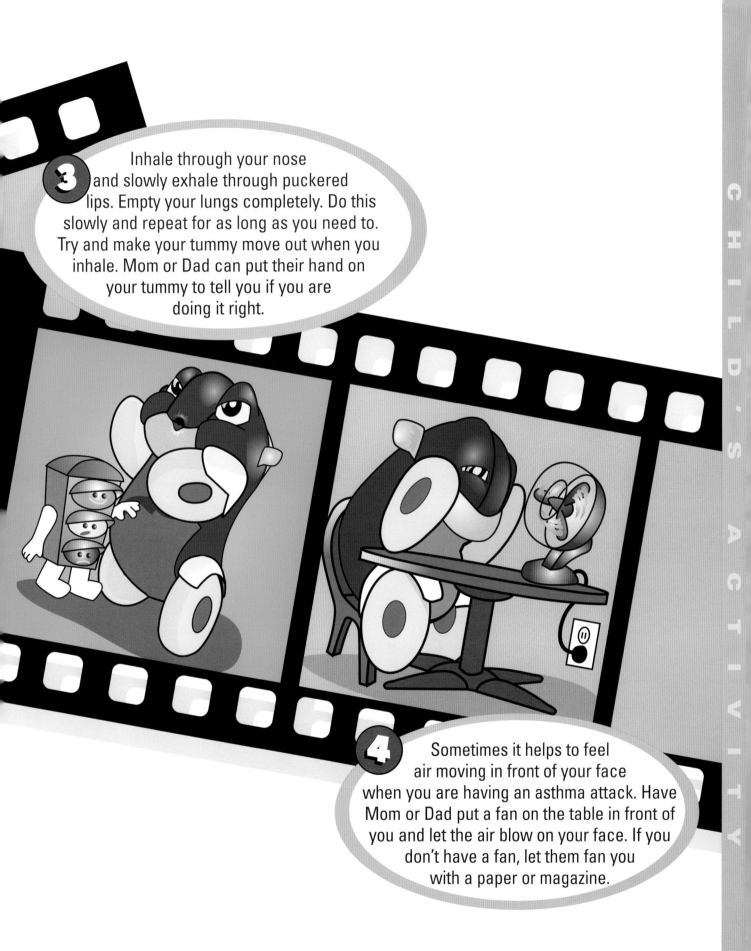

3 Inhale through your nose and slowly exhale through puckered lips. Empty your lungs completely. Do this slowly and repeat for as long as you need to. Try and make your tummy move out when you inhale. Mom or Dad can put their hand on your tummy to tell you if you are doing it right.

4 Sometimes it helps to feel air moving in front of your face when you are having an asthma attack. Have Mom or Dad put a fan on the table in front of you and let the air blow on your face. If you don't have a fan, let them fan you with a paper or magazine.

Section X Summary

SECTION X - STRESS AND RELAXATION

1. Medical research has demonstrated that extreme emotion such as crying and laughing may sometimes trigger an asthma attack.

2. The following steps can lessen the panic associated with an asthma attack:
- Taking your rescue medications.
- Sitting in a chair and leaning over a table on your elbows.
- Inhaling slowly through your nose and exhaling through puckered lips.
- Blowing a fan in your face to feel air movement.
- Remaining calm.

NOTES

_____

_____

_____

_____

_____

_____

_____

_____

_____

_____

_____

Asthma Treatment Plan

*T*he plan is based on the three asthma zones. Your child's zone is based on his peak flow readings and the absence or presence of asthma symptoms:

GREEN ZONE

Go!
- Symptom free
- Peak flow is greater than 80% of personal best

YELLOW ZONE

Caution!
- Asthma symptoms may be occurring
- Peak flow is between 50% and 80% of personal best

RED ZONE

Medical Emergency!
- Asthma symptoms are severe: coughing, wheezing, shortness of breath
- Peak flow is less than 50% of personal best

The treatment plan is designed to give you a step-by-step approach to managing your child's asthma on an ongoing, daily basis. If the plan does not keep your child in the green zone the majority of time, you need to notify your child's doctor. He may need to adjust the type or dose of medicine your child takes.

Included in the asthma treatment plan green zone is a section on exercise medicines. Your child's doctor may have prescribed daily medicines, considered to be controllers for the prevention of exercise-induced bronchospasm, or he may have prescribed a rescue type medicine to be used just before an exercise session. If you aren't sure about this area of your child's treatment plan, speak with his doctor to determine what type of treatment will best meet your child's needs.

It is a good idea to keep the asthma treatment plan in an obvious place for quick reference in an emergency. Good places include on the refrigerator or a family bulletin board. Make sure to review the plan with all your child's caregivers, making copies of the treatment plan for the daycare center, the school nurse, babysitters, and other relatives. Take a copy with you when you go on vacation.

The goal of the asthma treatment plan is to keep your child in the green zone. If you use the plan with the other information you have learned, including minimizing environmental triggers, increasing physical activity, eating a well-balanced diet, and managing stress and anxiety, your child will learn how to cope with his asthma without symptoms. We are providing you with three blank treatment plans for future changes or updates made by your child's doctor.

NOW THAT YOU'VE LEARNED ALL ABOUT YOUR CHILD'S ASTHMA, IT IS TIME TO DEVELOP HIS TREATMENT PLAN. THIS NEEDS TO BE WRITTEN BY YOUR CHILD'S DOCTOR OR ASTHMA EDUCATOR. THIS IS THE FINAL TOOL TO HELP YOU PULL TOGETHER ALL OF THE ELEMENTS AND BEGIN TAKING CONTROL OF YOUR CHILD'S FUTURE HEALTH.

ASTHMA TREATMENT PLAN

GREEN ZONE • No asthma symptoms
• Peak flow > 80% of Personal Best (Personal Best X .8 = _____)

1. Take controller medicine(s) on a daily basis.

MEDICINE	AMOUNT	HOW OFTEN
1.		
2.		

2. Take other medicines prescribed by the doctor (i.e., antihistamines, decongestants, nasal sprays, bronchodilators).

MEDICINE	AMOUNT	HOW OFTEN
1.		
2.		
3.		
4.		

3. Take medicines for exercise (if separate from controllers).

MEDICINE	AMOUNT	HOW OFTEN
1.		
2.		

NOTE: If your child is using rescue medicines more than twice per week (not including use for exercise), you must notify your child's doctor. The controllers are not helping your child's asthma stay in this zone.

YELLOW ZONE • Asthma symptoms may be occurring
• Peak flow between _____ and _____. (Personal Best X .5 and Personal Best X.8)

1. Start rescue medicine(s):

MEDICINE	AMOUNT	HOW OFTEN
1.		
2.		

2. Increase or add controller medicine(s):

MEDICINE	AMOUNT	HOW OFTEN
1.		
2.		
3.		
4.		

3. Eliminate physical activity and exercise until your child returns to the green zone.

4. After the peak flow is greater than _____ (80% of Personal Best) and symptoms stop, maintain the yellow zone treatment plan for _____ days.

5. If peak flow remains between _____ and _____ (50% to 80% of Personal Best) and symptoms persist for greater than 24 hours, notify your child's doctor.

RED ZONE • Asthma symptoms are severe. They may include coughing, wheezing and/or shortness of breath.
• Peak flow less than _____ (Personal Best X .5) or your child cannot perform a peak flow.

1. Start rescue medicine(s). Repeat medicine every 20 minutes X 3.

MEDICINE	AMOUNT	HOW OFTEN
1.		
2.		

2. Start oral steroids:

MEDICINE	AMOUNT	HOW OFTEN
1.		

3. Immediate medical attention is necessary. Notify your child's doctor.

4. If symptoms lessen and peak flows return to the yellow zone, follow the yellow zone treatment plan and notify your child's doctor.

Emergency: 911   Dr. _____   Hospital _____

ASTHMA TREATMENT PLAN

GREEN ZONE • No asthma symptoms
• Peak flow > 80% of Personal Best (Personal Best X .8 = _____)

1. Take controller medicine(s) on a daily basis.

MEDICINE	AMOUNT	HOW OFTEN
1.		
2.		

2. Take other medicines prescribed by the doctor (i.e., antihistamines, decongestants, nasal sprays, bronchodilators).

MEDICINE	AMOUNT	HOW OFTEN
1.		
2.		
3.		
4.		

3. Take medicines for exercise (if separate from controllers).

MEDICINE	AMOUNT	HOW OFTEN
1.		
2.		

NOTE: If your child is using rescue medicines more than twice per week (not including use for exercise), you must notify your child's doctor. The controllers are not helping your child's asthma stay in this zone.

YELLOW ZONE • Asthma symptoms may be occurring
• Peak flow between _____ and _____. (Personal Best X .5 and Personal Best X.8)

1. Start rescue medicine(s):

MEDICINE	AMOUNT	HOW OFTEN
1.		
2.		

2. Increase or add controller medicine(s):

MEDICINE	AMOUNT	HOW OFTEN
1.		
2.		
3.		
4.		

3. Eliminate physical activity and exercise until your child returns to the green zone.

4. After the peak flow is greater than _____ (80% of Personal Best) and symptoms stop, maintain the yellow zone treatment plan for _____ days.

5. If peak flow remains between _____ and _____ (50% to 80% of Personal Best) and symptoms persist for greater than 24 hours, notify your child's doctor.

RED ZONE • Asthma symptoms are severe. They may include coughing, wheezing and/or shortness of breath.
• Peak flow less than _____ (Personal Best X .5) or your child cannot perform a peak flow.

1. Start rescue medicine(s). Repeat medicine every 20 minutes X 3.

MEDICINE	AMOUNT	HOW OFTEN
1.		
2.		

2. Start oral steroids:

MEDICINE	AMOUNT	HOW OFTEN
1.		

3. Immediate medical attention is necessary. Notify your child's doctor.

4. If symptoms lessen and peak flows return to the yellow zone, follow the yellow zone treatment plan and notify your child's doctor.

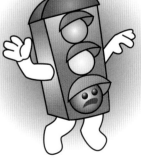

Emergency: 911   Dr. _____   Hospital _____   **93**

P A R E N T   P A G E - S E C T I O N   X I

GREEN ZONE • No asthma symptoms
• Peak flow > 80% of Personal Best (Personal Best X .8 = _____)

1. Take controller medicine(s) on a daily basis.

MEDICINE	AMOUNT	HOW OFTEN
1.		
2.		

2. Take other medicines prescribed by the doctor (i.e., antihistamines, decongestants, nasal sprays, bronchodilators).

MEDICINE	AMOUNT	HOW OFTEN
1.		
2.		
3.		
4.		

NOTE: If your child is using rescue medicines more than twice per week (not including use for exercise), you must notify your child's doctor. The controllers are not helping your child's asthma stay in this zone.

3. Take medicines for exercise (if separate from controllers).

MEDICINE	AMOUNT	HOW OFTEN
1.		
2.		

YELLOW ZONE • Asthma symptoms may be occurring
• Peak flow between _____ and _____ . (Personal Best X .5 and Personal Best X.8)

1. Start rescue medicine(s):

MEDICINE	AMOUNT	HOW OFTEN
1.		
2.		

2. Increase or add controller medicine(s):

MEDICINE	AMOUNT	HOW OFTEN
1.		
2.		
3.		
4.		

3. Eliminate physical activity and exercise until your child returns to the green zone.

4. After the peak flow is greater than _____ (80% of Personal Best) and symptoms stop, maintain the yellow zone treatment plan for _____ days.

5. If peak flow remains between _____ and _____ (50% to 80% of Personal Best) and symptoms persist for greater than 24 hours, notify your child's doctor.

RED ZONE • Asthma symptoms are severe. They may include coughing, wheezing and/or shortness of breath.
• Peak flow less than _____ (Personal Best X .5) or your child cannot perform a peak flow.

1. Start rescue medicine(s). Repeat medicine every 20 minutes X 3.

MEDICINE	AMOUNT	HOW OFTEN
1.		
2.		

2. Start oral steroids:

MEDICINE	AMOUNT	HOW OFTEN
1.		

3. Immediate medical attention is necessary. Notify your child's doctor.

4. If symptoms lessen and peak flows return to the yellow zone, follow the yellow zone treatment plan and notify your child's doctor.

Emergency: 911   Dr. _____   Hospital _____

You and Zoey have learned so much!

You can live a happy and healthy life, even with asthma. On the next page, Zoey gives you your reminders for controlling your asthma.

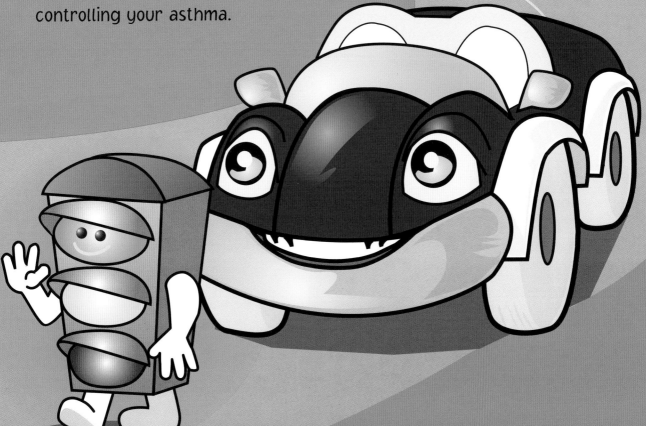

95

Remember 4 things to stay in your Green Zone

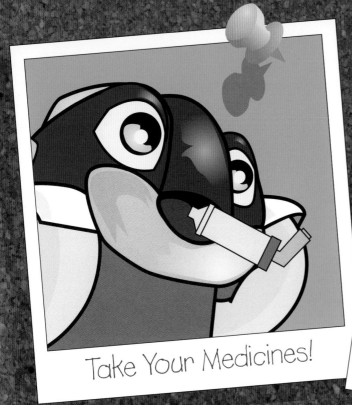

Take Your Medicines!

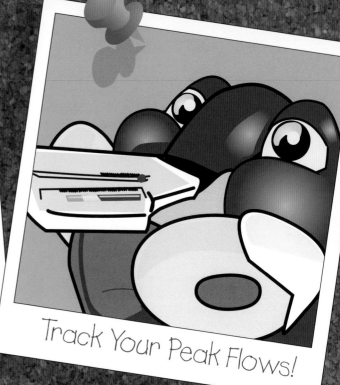

Track Your Peak Flows!

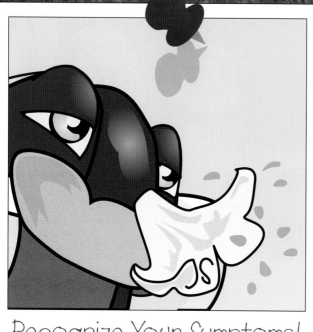

Recognize Your Symptoms!

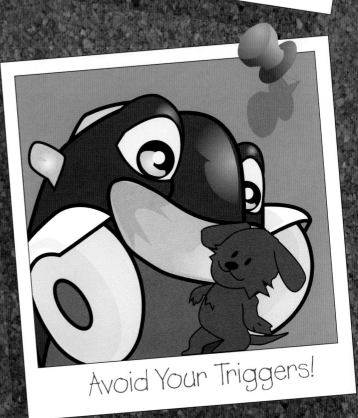

Avoid Your Triggers!

CHILD'S ACTIVITY

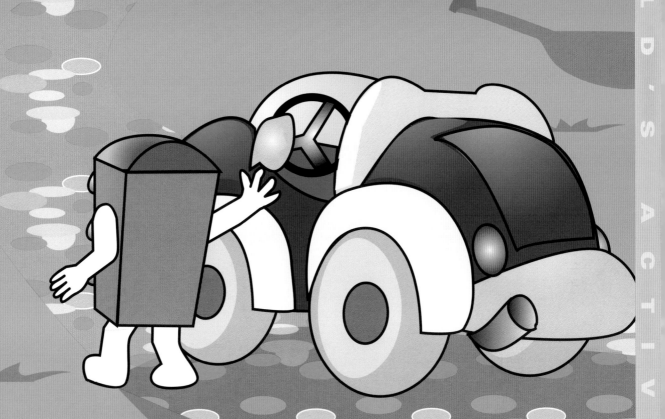

The End

Section XI Summary

SECTION XI - ASTHMA TREATMENT PLAN

1. The asthma treatment plan should keep your child in their green zone the majority of the time.

2. All of the following should have copies of your child's asthma treatment plan:
- Home
- School
- Relatives
- Babysitter or Day Care

3. The asthma treatment plan should be updated whenever there is a change in medications or the personal best peak flow number.

NOTES

_____

_____

_____

_____

_____

_____

_____

_____

_____

_____

References

Zoey L.P.
1759 Grandstand
San Antonio, TX 78238
1-866-275-9639
www.zoeyzones.com

American Lung Association
1740 Broadway
New York, NY 10019
www.lungusa.org

Asthma and Allergy Foundation
of America
1125 15th Street, North West, Suite 502
Washington, D.C. 20005
1-800-727-8462
www.aafa.org

National Asthma Education
and Prevention Program
National Heart, Lung and Blood Institute
P.O. Box 30105
Bethesda, MD 20824-0105
www.nih.gov

Allergy and Asthma Network/Mothers
of Asthmatics, Inc.
3554 Chain Bridge Rd., Ste 200
Fairfax, VA 22030-2709
1-800-878-4403
www.mothersofasthmatics.org

American Academy of Allergy, Asthma
and Immunology
(Physician Referral Line)
611 East Wells Street
Milwaukee, WI 53202
1-800-822-2762
www.aaaai.org

American College of Allergy, Asthma
and Immunology
85 West Algonquin Road
Arlington Heights, IL 60005
www.allergy.mcg.edu

National Jewish Medical and
Research Center
1400 Jackson Street
Denver, CO 80206
1-800-423-8891
www.nationaljewish.org

OTHER ASTHMA BOOKS

American Academy of Pediatrics Guide to
Your Child's Allergies and Asthma:
Breathing Easy and Bringing up Healthy,
Active Children
by Michael J. Welch, M.D., American
Academy of Pediatrics
2000, ISBN: 067976982X

Children with Asthma: A Manual
for Parents
by Thomas F. Plaut,
Carla Brennan (Illustrator)
1998, ISBN: 0914625217

Relieve The Squeeze: How to Take Control
of Your Asthma
by Peggy Guthart Strauss
Photographs by Lucy Dahl
2000, ISBN: 0670893390

Taking Asthma to School
(Special Kids in Schools Series, No 2)
by Kim Gosselin, et al
1998, ISBN: 1891383019

The ABC's of Asthma: An Asthma
Alphabet Book for Kids of All Ages
by Kim Gosselin, et al
1998, ISBN: 1891383043

The American Lung Association Family
Guide to Asthma and Allergies: How You
and Your Children Can Breathe Easier
by The American Lung Advisory Group,
Norman Edelman (Contributor)
1998, ISBN: 0316036156

Weaver's Daughter
by Kimberly Brubaker Bradley
2000, ISBN: 0385327692

*Some branches of the American Lung
Association offer summer asthma camps for
children. Contact your local chapter of the
American Lung Association to find an
asthma camp near you. Or, go to Zoey's
website at www.zoeyzones.com to get a
comprehensive list of asthma camps
throughout the USA.*

REFERENCES

Glossary

A

aerosol: small particles in a gas or air. A gas under pressure that contains medicine which is breathed into the lungs.

airways: a series of small tubes inside the lungs that allow air to be breathed in and out.

allergen: a foreign substance that can cause an allergic response in the body but is only harmful to some people.

allergy: condition in which the body has an immune reaction to a normally harmless substance.

animal dander: dry scales shed from the skin or hair of animals, or the feathers of birds.

anticholinergic: a rescue medicine that lessens muscle spasm of the airways, used commonly by people that suffer from severe asthma attacks or those that cannot tolerate short-acting bronchodilators.

asthma: a chronic inflammatory disease of the airways in the lungs, characterized by attacks of wheezing, coughing, shortness of breath, and chest tightness. There may also be increased mucous production in the lungs during attacks.

asthma educator: a healthcare worker specifically trained to teach people with asthma how to control and manage their disease. Common asthma educators include respiratory therapists, nurses, and pharmacists.

asthma severity: a classification system used to determine how mild or severe a person's asthma is. The classification is determined before the person begins taking asthma medicines.

asthma treatment plan: a step-wise, daily approach to managing asthma and responding to the three zones which are based on the presence or absence of symptoms and peak flow readings.

asthma zones: the three asthma zones: green, yellow, and red which are determined by peak flow readings and the absence or presence of symptoms.

attack: a dramatic term for an asthma episode with increased symptoms and decreased peak flow readings.

B

beta-blocker: a medicine commonly found in heart medications and some eye drops or ointments.

bronchodilator: a medicine used to relax contractions of the airways to improve breathing.

bronchospasm: an abnormal contraction of the airways, resulting in narrowing and blockage.

C

chest tightness: a symptom of an asthma episode where the person experiences a tight feeling in the chest or lungs.

chronic illness: a disease or disorder that develops slowly and persists for a long time. It can sometimes remain for a person's lifetime.

compliance: adherence to the asthma treatment plan as prescribed by the doctor.

controller medication: daily medicine used to prevent or reduce the frequency and severity of asthma attacks.

corticosteroid: a steroid or cortisone-like medicine used to reduce the swelling of the airways.

coughing: a sudden, forceful release of air from the lungs. It clears the lungs and throats of irritants and fluids. It is a common symptom of asthma.

D

Diskus: a brand name for a dry powder inhaler device.

dust mites: microscopic bugs found in dust particles. A common trigger for attacks in most people with asthma.

E

episode: a period of time when there is a presence of asthma symptoms, a decrease in peak flow reading, and the need for additional asthma medicine.

exacerbation: a worsening in the seriousness of the asthma.

exercise-induced asthma: a form of asthma in which the trigger for an attack is exercise or play.

F

FEV1: the amount of air that a person can forcefully exhale in one second. It is a measurement obtained during a pulmonary function test to determine the status of the large and small airways inside the lungs.

G

gastroesophageal reflux: a backflow of stomach contents into the esophagus or food tube. It may cause irritation that leads to bronchospasm.

green zone: an asthma zone in which the person is experiencing no symptoms and their peak flow is greater than 80% of their personal best.

H

holding chamber: a device used with a metered dose inhaler that holds the medicine mist, allowing the user to get more medicine into their lungs. Also known as a spacer.

I

indoor pollutant: irritant found inside a building that may be a trigger for an asthma attack. Common indoor pollutants include dust, mold, strong fragrances, chemical odors, tobacco smoke, and fireplace smoke.

inflammation: a swelling response of the tissues in the body to irritants or triggers.

inhaled corticosteroid: medicine that is inhaled to prevent swelling of the airways and reduce inflammation that already exists. It is the most effective type of controller medicine used for people with persistent asthma.

L

leukotriene modifier: a group of controller medicines that work by blocking the formation or action of leukotrienes in the airways, thereby blocking part of an asthma reaction.

long-acting bronchodilator: a slow-released or sustained-released medicine used as a controller medicine to prevent bronchospasm, particularly at night and with exercise.

long-term control medicine: medicine taken daily on a long-term basis to control and prevent asthma symptoms of people with any form of persistent asthma.

lungs: a pair of light, spongy organs in the chest, which are the main part of the body's breathing system.

M

MDI dose counter: a device placed on a metered dose inhaler to count the number of doses used.

metered dose inhaler (MDI): a device that turns liquid medicine into an aerosol mist that is inhaled into the lungs.

methylxanthines: a group of controller medicines that provide moderate bronchodilation for nighttime symptoms. It includes the drug theophylline.

mild intermittent asthma: a classification of asthma severity in which asthma symptoms are less than twice per week, nighttime symptoms are less that twice per month, attacks are infrequent and/or brief, physical activity is generally normal, and the FEV1 is 80% or greater than predicted.

101

mild persistent asthma: a classification of asthma severity in which asthma symptoms occur more than twice per week, but less than once per day, nighttime symptoms occur three to four times per month, attacks occur less than twice per week, physical activity is sometimes decreased, and the FEV1 is 80% or greater than predicted.

moderate persistent asthma: a classification of asthma severity in which asthma symptoms occur daily, physical activity is decreased, attacks occur more than twice per week, nighttime symptoms occur more than once per week, and the FEV1 is between 60% and 80% of predicted.

N

nasal corticosteroid: a liquid, cortisone-like medicine that is sprayed into the nasal passages to prevent or reduce swelling and congestion that may result from chronic rhinitis, sinusitis, or exposure to allergens.

National Institutes of Health (NIH): a government health agency that has various groups of medical specialists that research, formulate, write, and publish standards of care for the treatment of various chronic diseases.

nebulizer circuit: a plastic circuit that is comprised of tubing that attaches to a nebulizer compressor, a medicine cup to hold the liquid medicine, and a mouthpiece or mask that the patient breathes through. It changes the liquid medicine into an aerosol mist that can be inhaled into the lungs.

nebulizer compressor: the air compressor unit used to turn the liquid medicine in a nebulizer circuit into an aerosol mist. It can be electric or battery operated.

nighttime symptom: an asthma symptom such as wheezing, coughing, shortness of breath, or chest tightness that occur at night and awaken a person from sleep.

non-steroidal anti-inflammatory medicine: a group of controller medicines that are milder than corticosteroids and often used in small children, or to prevent symptoms associated with exercise and exposure to known allergens. They include the drugs cromolyn sodium and nedocromil.

O

obstructive lung disease: any blockage of the breathing tract that may be linked to symptoms of swelling in the airways.

outdoor allergen: a foreign substance that acts as an irritant or trigger for persons with allergic sensitivity to the substance. Common outdoor allergens include grasses, trees and shrubs, pollen, and mold.

outdoor pollutant: irritant that is found outside in the environment and may trigger an asthma attack. Common outdoor pollutants are air pollution or smog, smoke, or exhaust fumes.

P

panic: a strong, sudden fear that causes terror, which may result in the inability to properly respond or react to the event.

peak flow diary: a daily log used to track peak flow results and asthma symptoms.

peak flow meter: a device used to measure peak expired flow rate (PEFR).

personal best peak flow: the highest peak flow score that a person can achieve when the airways are clear, asthma symptoms are absent, and their technique is good.

powdered dose inhaler: a device that allows for the inhalation of a powdered form of medicine into the lungs.

pulmonary function test (PFT): a test of the lungs and the ability of the person to move air in and out of their lungs through their airways.

Q

quick-relief medicine: another name for rescue medicine, used in the treatment of an asthma attack.

R

red zone: an asthma zone considered a medical emergency. The person is experiencing severe symptoms, breathing is difficult and the peak flow is less than 50% of their personal best. Rescue medicines are used and outside medical assistance may be necessary.

rescue medicine: a group of medicines used to provide relief of bronchospasm, coughing, wheezing, and shortness of breath during an asthma attack. This group includes the short-acting bronchodilators, anticholinergics, and systemic corticosteroids.

respiratory tract infection: any infectious disease of the upper or lower breathing tract.

rhinitis: a swelling of the mucous membranes of the nose, with a nasal discharge.

S

severe persistent asthma: a classification of asthma severity in which the symptoms are continuous, nighttime symptoms are frequent, physical activity is very limited, attacks occur frequently, and the FEV1 is less than 60% of predicted.

short-acting bronchodilator: a bronchodilator that relaxes the smooth muscle of the airways during a bronchospasm. They usually provide relief within 30 minutes of use. They are the most effective medicine available to relieve bronchospasm and are frequently used before exercise to prevent exercise-induced asthma.

shortness of breath: a feeling of breathlessness or difficulty in breathing.

sinusitis: a swelling of one or more nasal sinus cavities that may be a complication of a respiratory infection, dental infection, allergy, a change in atmospheric pressure, or a defect of the nose.

spacer: a device used with a metered dose inhaler that provides a chamber between the MDI and mouth for a more effective dose of medicine. Also known as a holding chamber.

sulfite sensitivity: a sensitivity to foods that contain sulfites, preservatives used in processing of beer, wine, dried fruit, instant potatoes, processed meats and Asian foods that contain MSG.

symptom: anything you feel or notice that is different from usual; for example, shortness of breath, coughing, or wheezing.

systemic corticosteroid: a corticosteroid that is taken internally that affects the whole body rather than a single part of the body. In asthma, this is a group of rescue medicines that are normally used for severe asthma episodes for a short period of time.

T

trigger: an instigator or precipitating factor that causes airway swelling and asthma symptoms.

W

wheezing: a whistling sound in the throat marked by a high-pitched, musical quality. It is caused by a high flow of air through a narrowed airway. It may be heard during inspiration or exhalation, or both.

Y

yellow zone: an asthma zone where a person is experiencing moderate symptoms, their peak flow is between 50% and 80% of their personal best, and additional medicines are needed.

Index

Visit our Zoey Store on our website at
www.zoeyzones.com
to order any of the following items.

Or call us toll free at
1-866-ASK-ZOEY

- **Zoey and the Zones**™
  A Story for Children with Asthma

- **Zoey and the Zones**™
  Companion Workbook for Parents of Children with Asthma

- Zoey Coloring Book

- Zoey Posters

- Zoey Game

- Zoey Medic Alert Jewelry

- Asthma Treatment Plans

- Peak Flow Diary

- Pillow and Mattress Covers

- Zoey and Light Buddy Beanie Toys

- Zoey Newsletter Subscription

- Zoey Peak Flow Meters

- Zoey Masks for Nebulizers and Spacers

ADDITIONAL PRODUCTS

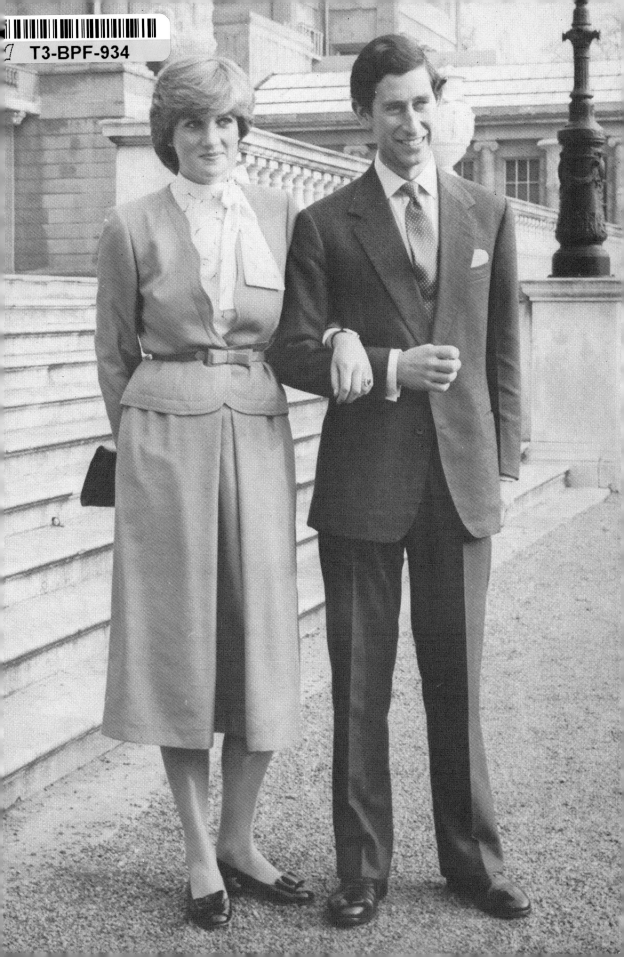

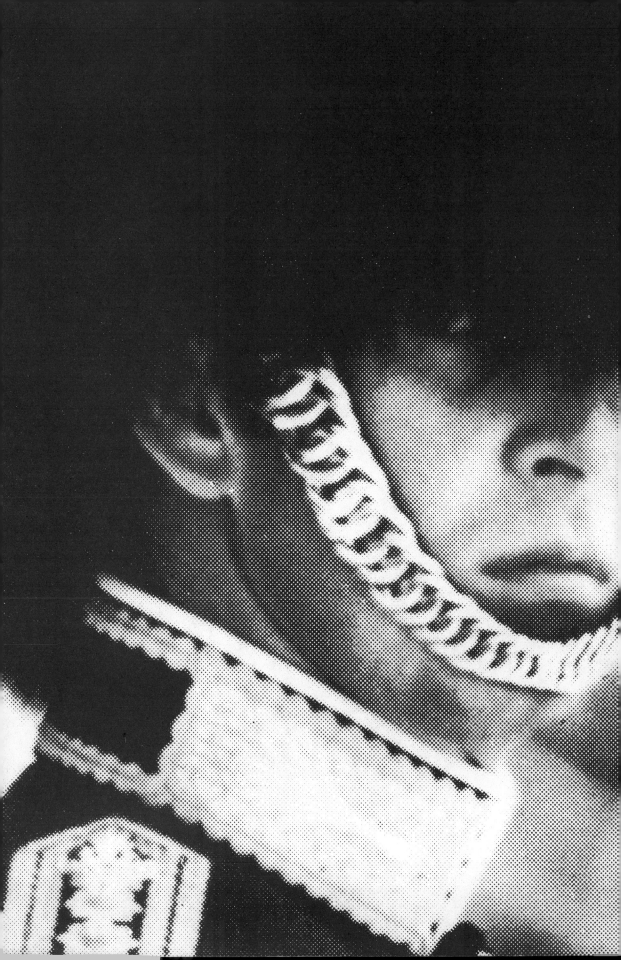

Charles
In His
Own
Words.

Compiled by Rosemary York.
Designed by Perry Neville.

New York · London

Published 1981 by Omnibus Press
(a division of Book Sales Limited).

Book concept, design & origination:
Perry Neville.
Design assistant: Gill Lockhart.
Picture research: Susan Ready.
Original series styling: Pearce Marchbank.
Cover photograph: Camera Press/Les Wilson.

ISBN: 0-8256-3954-9
Order No. 030954

Typeset by G.W.Young Photosetters Limited,
Brighton Road, Surbiton, Surrey.

Printed in the U.S.A.

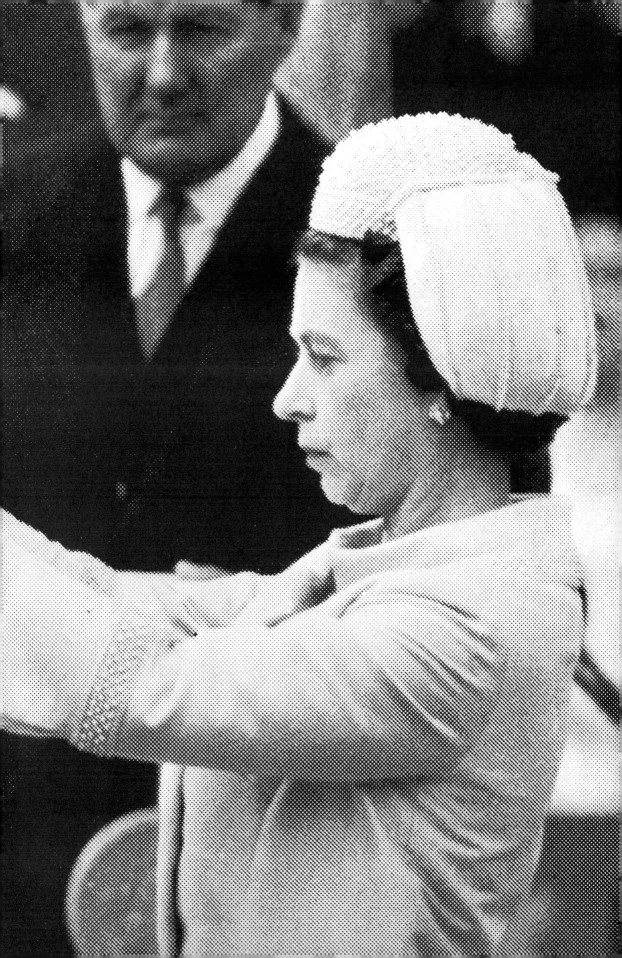

Prince Charles is a favourite of the Press and has been the subject of many "official" biographies.

He has only to fall from a horse or remark on a pretty girl to make the front page – not just in Britain, but throughout the world.

From the announcement of his birth to his choice of a fairytale princess, his whole life has been recorded and photographed without mercy. Yet, he talks very little about himself and rarely gives interviews.

Here his comments, thoughts and humour on almost every subject have been selected from the archives of newspapers, radio and television and collected together for the first time. He talks about school, his family and the problems of making friends, his hobbies, sports and, of course, his marriage.

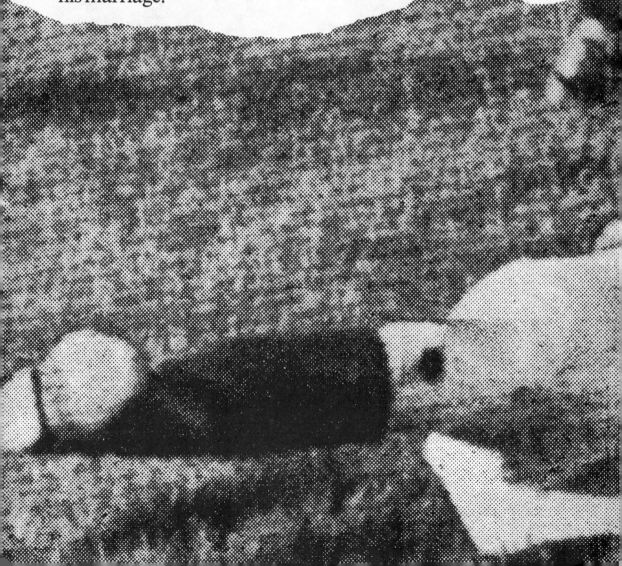

Charles In His Own Words presents a composite picture of the private individual behind the public myth. He emerges as a Twentieth Century prince with a modest, witty and perceptive view of the world. *Rosemary York.*

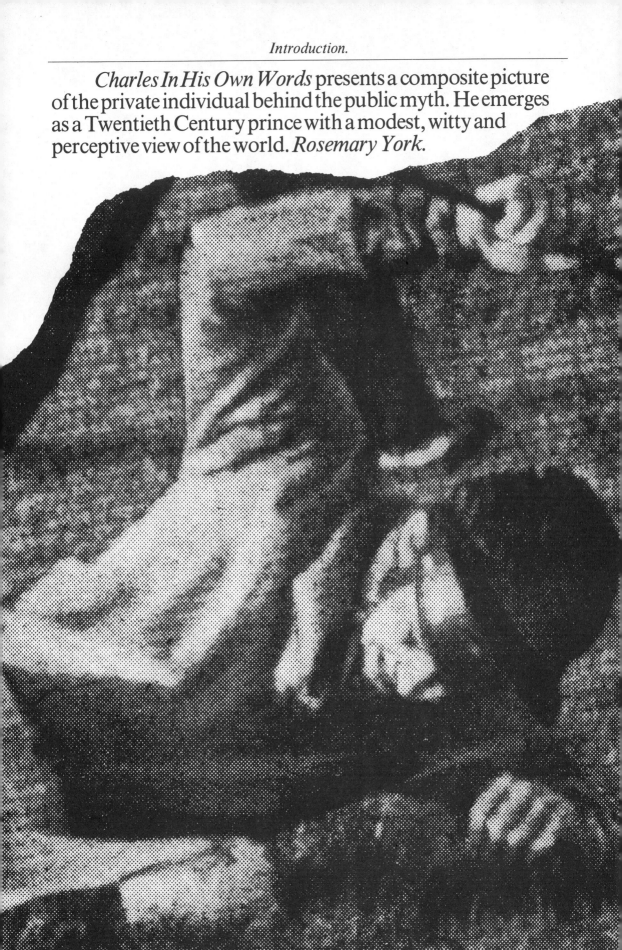

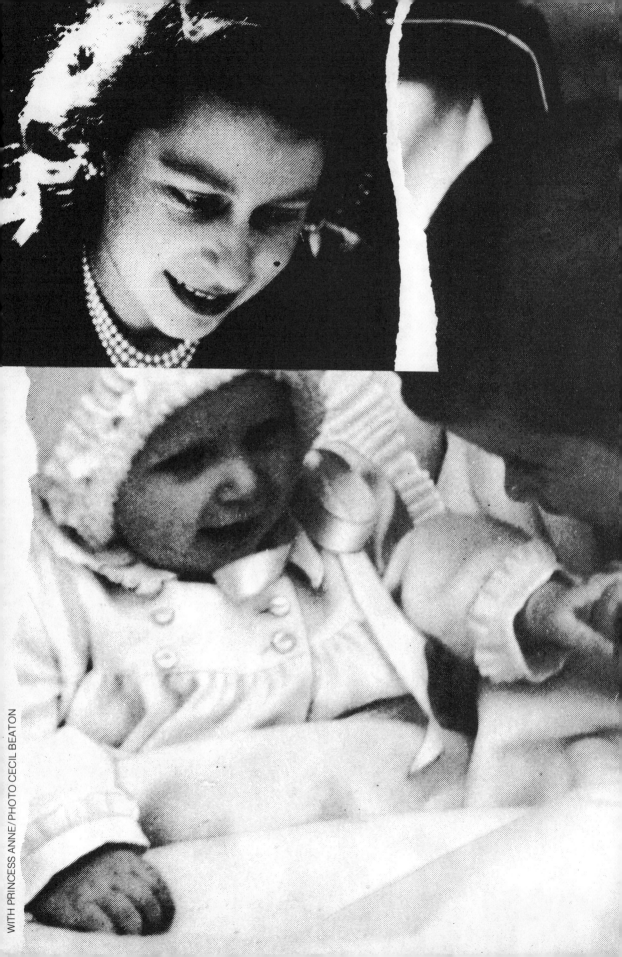

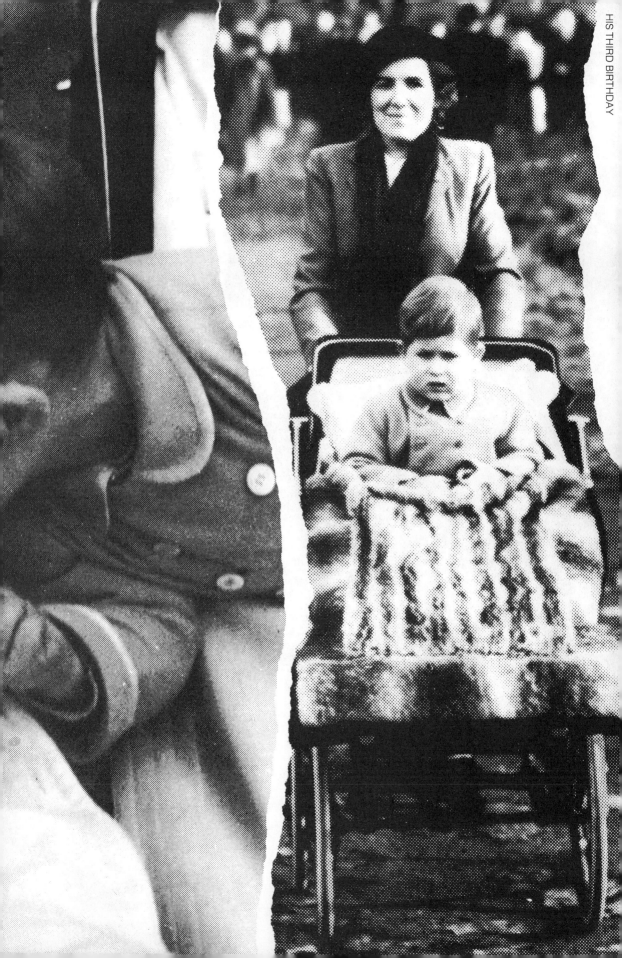

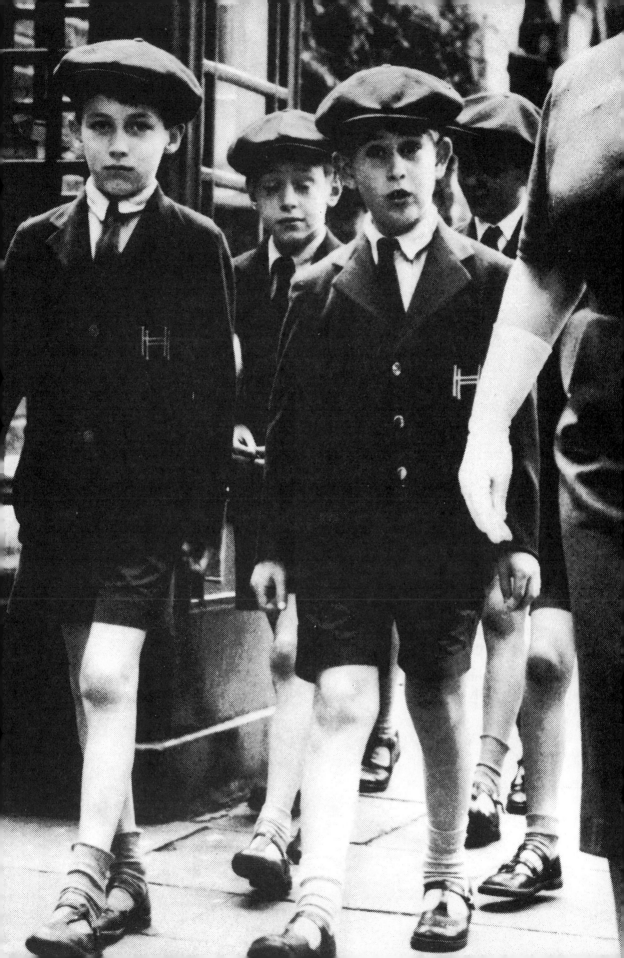

Schooldays.

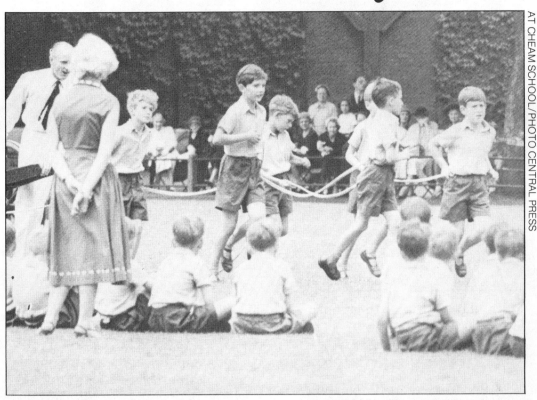

Mummy, what *are* schoolboys? (Age 8)

Charles went first to Hill House, then Cheam, and eventually to Gordonstoun:

I suppose I could have gone to the local comprehensive or the local grammar, but I'm not sure it would have done me much good. I think a public school gives you a great deal of self-discipline and experience and responsibility, and it is the responsibility which is so worthwhile.

It's very rewarding and it gives you the added confidence in yourself that you have the ability to do something for other people, and they trust you to do it. I think this is very important.

You learn the way they say the monkey learns: watching its parents! On the whole, you pick it up as you go along.

I did some constitutional history when I was at school, but I didn't get very far with it. You can't teach children a great deal of such a complicated and sophisticated subject by making them read books or write essays. After school, I had to do so many other things that there wasn't time or need to get down to it as I would have liked.

That's the advantage of meeting a number of people who know a lot about it, and talking to them. The Lord Chancellor, for instance. Now I'm going to have more time in this country, I'm going to try to learn more about it.

I wasn't made to follow in my father's footsteps in any sense or in any way. His attitude was very simple: he told me what were the pros and cons of all the possibilities and what he thought was best. Then he left me to decide.

I freely subjected myself to what he thought best because I saw how wise he

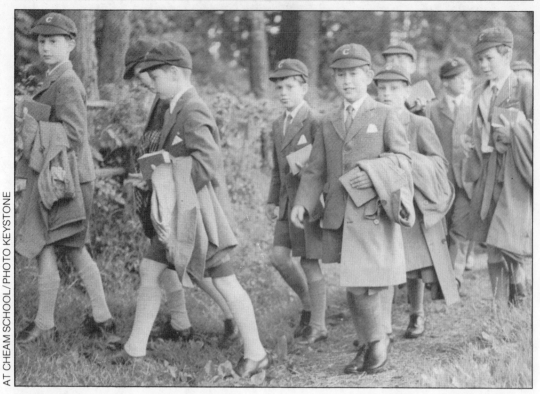

AT CHEAM SCHOOL/ PHOTO KEYSTONE

was. By the time I had to be educated, I had perfect confidence in my father's judgement.

When children are young, of course, you have to decide for them. I'm talking about the later stage when they are old enough to share in decisions about themselves.

Gordonstoun.

I'm glad I went to Gordonstoun. It wasn't the toughness of the place – that's all much exaggerated by reports – it was the general character of the education there. Kurt Hahn's principles provide an education which tries to balance the physical and mental, with an emphasis on self-reliance to develop a rounded human being.

I didn't enjoy school as much as I might have, but that was only because I'm happier at home than anywhere else.

Gordonstoun developed my will-power and self-control. It helped me to discipline myself, and I think that discipline, not in the sense of making you bath in cold water, but in the Latin sense – giving shape and form and tidiness to your

life – is the most important thing your education can do.

Dr. Kurt Hahn, the founder, did not exactly require boys to undergo initiation ceremonies, but believed that a boy must challenge himself and discover his own level of endurance and will-power. He believed in the acquisition of self-knowledge and self-discipline.

My experience was that this worked surprisingly well and that's why I'm so keen that others should experience it.

I'm always astonished by the amount of rot that is talked about Gordonstoun and the careless use of ancient clichés to describe it. It was only tough in that it demanded more from you as an individual, mentally and physically, than most other schools.

I believe it taught me a great deal about myself and my own abilities and disabilities, and it taught me to take challenges and initiatives.

At my school we went in for "adventure." We ran our own fire brigade, we had our own sea rescue service, mountain rescue, surf life-saving, coastguard, etc. It *was* adventure. And we were damn good. We used to say that the reason why the local fire brigade sometimes didn't call us out was because we were better than they were.

On the problems of making friends at school:

At Gordonstoun, you could hear them accusing other people of sucking-up and this is a problem. But it's one of those things that you learn through experience – how to sense who are the ones who are sucking-up, and who are being genuine.

Of course the trouble is, that very often, the worst people come first and the really nice people hang back because they don't want to be accused of sucking-up.

On a school trip round the Hebrides, fourteen-year-old Charles drank an illegal glass of brandy in a hotel bar. The incident made front page news around the world:

Well, I thought it was the end of the earth. I was all ready to pack my bags and leave for Siberia.

We went to Stornoway and I went to a hotel to have a meal. While we were waiting for a table, a lot of people were looking in the windows, so I thought,

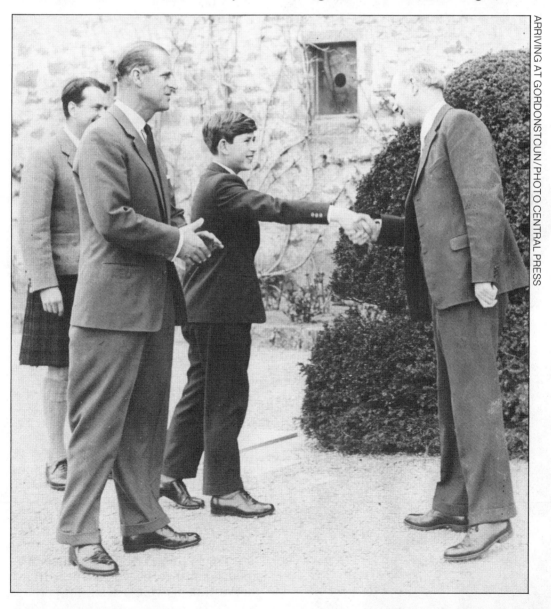

ARRIVING AT GORDONSTOUN/PHOTO CENTRAL PRESS

"I can't bear this any more," and went off somewhere else. The only other place was the bar.

Having never been into a bar before, the first thing I thought of doing was having a drink, of course. It seemed the most sensible thing. And being terrified, not knowing what to do, I said the first drink that came into my head, which happened to be cherry brandy, because I'd drunk it before, when it was cold, out shooting.

Hardly had I taken a sip when the whole world exploded around my ears. That's all.

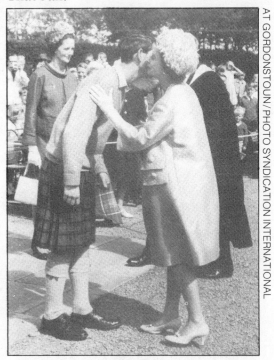

PHOTO SYNDICATION INTERNATIONAL

AT GORDONSTOUN/PHOTO SYNDICATION INTERNATIONAL

Timbertop.

Charles went to Timbertop School in Australia:

It was a very sad moment, of course, leaving England, seeing one's father and sister standing on the tarmac and waving goodbye. I found the moment I was in the air, it was much better. When I got to Australia, the people were so friendly and so welcoming.

I must admit I'd been apprehensive about going there because I'd heard that the Australians were critical and, perhaps,

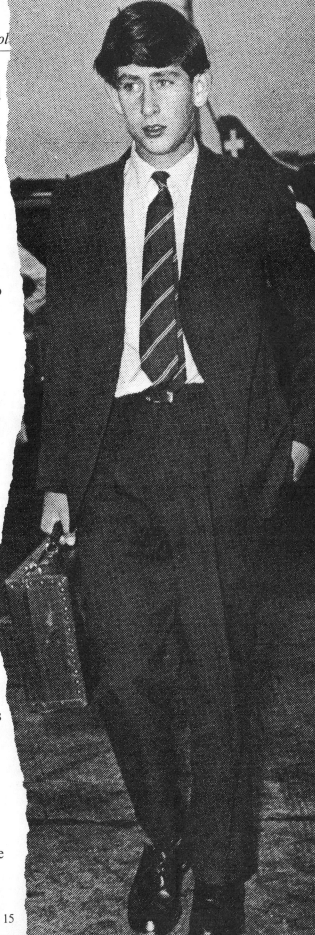

would show their feelings. I was worried about how I would appear to them, but after I'd been there an hour I found I'd had absolutely no need to worry.

The school is situated in the foothills of the Dividing Range and all the buildings are extraordinarily well hidden from view as there are gum-trees everywhere. The boys live in units, or bungalow-type buildings, of which there are nine, holding fifteen boys apiece.

The Chapel is in the centre and is in the shape of a continuous steep roof that reaches to the ground. Behind the altar, there is a huge window that looks out on to a series of ridges receding into the distance.

When I arrived here, everything was very dry and brown, but now it is all green since the early rains came.

I've been out to several farms in the area and have watched some shearing being done. I was asked to try my hand, but of course made rather a mess of it, and left a somewhat shredded sheep.

Everyone asks how Australia compares with England, which is a very difficult question, as there isn't really a comparison. The mountains are so different from Scotland because there are no ordered fields, but rolling hills covered in grass, with gum-trees dotted about everywhere.

I came over here expecting boiling weather all the time but one soon discovered one's error, as it can certainly become very cold, especially during winter, while it's summer term at Gordonstoun.

A popular cry seems to be that Timbertop is very similar to Gordonstoun.

From what I make of it, Timbertop is very individual. All the boys are virtually the same age, fourteen to fifteen; there are no prefects, and the masters do all the work that boys otherwise do in a school. This way, I think there is much more contact between masters and boys, as everyone is placed in the same sort of situation.

There is a lot of wood-chopping done here, but I'm afraid it's very essential as

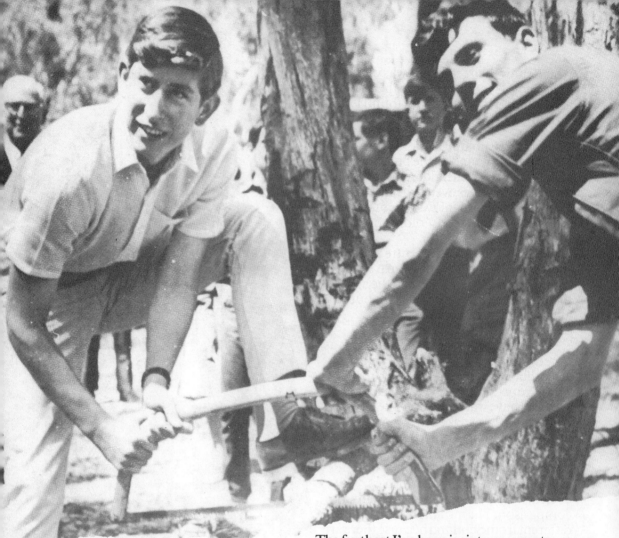

the boys' boilers have to be stoked with logs, and the kitchen uses a huge number. The first week I was here I was made to go out and chop up logs on a hillside in boiling hot weather. I could hardly see my hands for blisters after that!

You had to go on expeditions every weekend into the bush and you had two "cross-countries" a week. The first ones I had when I got there were absolutely horrifying. It was ninety degrees in the shade, with flies everywhere, and you sort of ran around amongst the kangaroos and things. Dust and everything.

Then one played fairly fierce games. They weren't organised games like football or anything like that: you chopped down trees.

Some boys managed to walk fantastic distances over a weekend of four days or less, covering up to two hundred miles.

The furthest I've been is sixty or seventy miles in three days, climbing about five peaks on the way. At the campsite, the cooking is done on an open fire in a trench. You have to be very careful in hot weather that you don't start a bush fire, and at the beginning of this term there was a total fire-ban in force, so we ate all the tinned food cold.

Apart from that, you virtually have to inspect every inch of ground ... in case there are ants or other ghastly creatures. There is one species called Bull Ants which are three-quarters of an inch long or more and they bite like mad!

In between all these diversions, work has to fit in somewhere. In fact, the weeks just seem to be a useful means of filling up the gaps between the weekends, which come round very quickly.

Obviously, work can't be taken quite as seriously as in an ordinary school, but there are classes all morning after Chapel

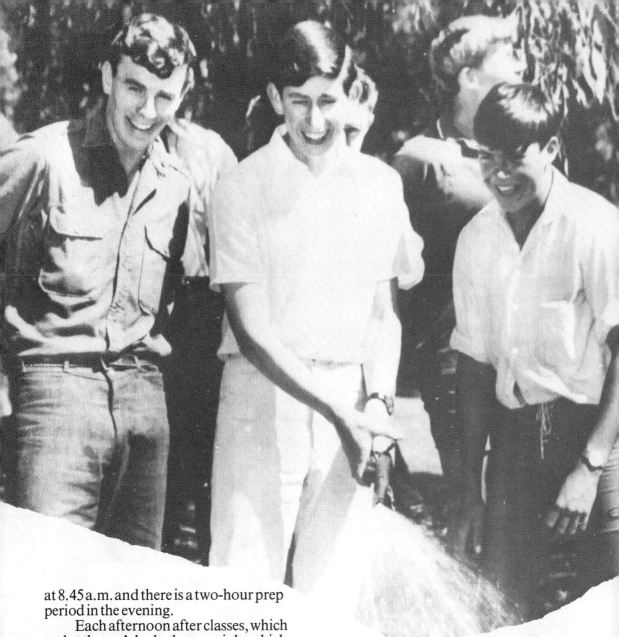

at 8.45 a.m. and there is a two-hour prep period in the evening.

Each afternoon after classes, which end at three o'clock, there are jobs which are rather equivalent to PW but involve chopping and splitting wood, feeding the pigs, cleaning out fly-traps (revolting glass bowls seething with flies and very ancient meat) or picking up bits of paper round the school.

There is no organised sport in the form of field games, but each Wednesday there is either a tug o' war between the boys' units, or houses, or, if it's hot, there is swimming or perhaps someone is feeling sufficiently cruel to organise a race that involves carrying half a tree for a certain distance.

I almost convinced one or two Australians outside the school that we rustled kangaroos at Timbertop and that we performed this art by creeping up on them from behind, grabbing them by the tail and flicking them over onto their backs, where you had them at your mercy.

More than any other experience, those years opened my eyes. You are judged there on how people see you and feel about you. There are no assumptions there. Having a title and being a member of the upper classes as often as not mitigates against you.

In Australia, you have to fend for yourself. I was fairly shy when I was

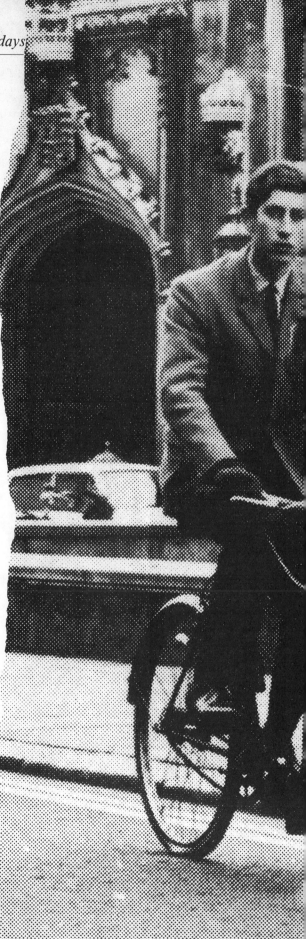

younger but Australia certainly cured me of that.

There may be limitations I have to accept, but not mixing isn't one of them. I do mix. It's one of the privileges of my position. If you say, "Well, you haven't lived with men who do this or that, or who haven't got this or that," I say, "Quite so, but I've *met* some of the people who live with them and do know about them – and that's more than many thousands of people in this country have the chance to do."

I absolutely adored it. I couldn't have enjoyed it more. The most wonderful experience I've ever had, I think.

That school's probably the reason why, whenever I come back to Australia, I experience a curious and inexplicable sensation that I belong.

Cambridge.

I'm one of those stupid bums who went to university. Well, I think it's helped me. You see, I really wanted to go to university because I felt that I hadn't had enough education at school, and I felt that going to university for another three years would round it off and give me just that much more.

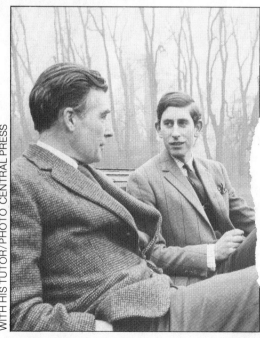

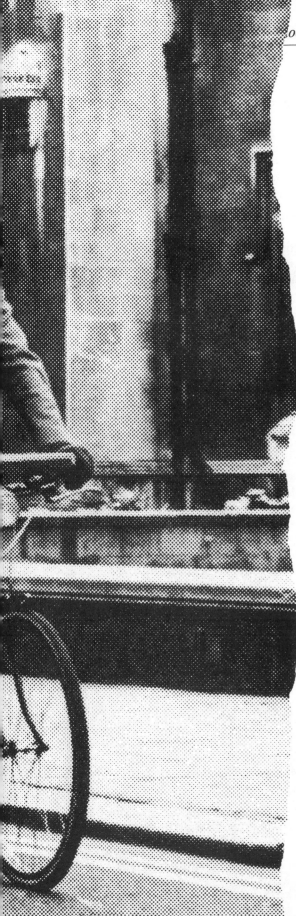

It would be marvellous to have three years when you are not bound by anything, not married, and haven't any particular job.

His first day at Trinity:

All I could see from the Mini on arrival were serried ranks of trousered legs, from which I had to distinguish those of the Master and the Senior Tutor.

My most vivid memory of that day is of several burly, bowler-hatted gentlemen (the College porters) dragging shut those magnificent wooden gates to prevent the crowd from following in. It was like a scene from the French Revolution.

Trinity means every modulation of light and weather, like the orange-pink glow from the stone of the Wren Library in the last rays from a wintry sun ... And the everlasting sound of photographers' boots ringing on the cobbles.

In the early morning, there is also the noise of the world coming to life beneath the window. This is something I find hard to accustom myself to, particularly the grinding noise of an Urban District Council dust lorry's engine rising and falling in spasmodic energy at seven o'clock in the morning accompanied by the jovial dustman's refrain of "O Come All Ye Faithful" and the headsplitting clang of the bins.

I've always been interested in history, even when I was quite small. I don't know whether it's me or being born into what I was, but I *feel* history. It fascinates me. I'm a romantic at heart, really.

At Gordonstoun I was very keen on it, and when the time came for me to go to Cambridge and choose my subjects, I thought, "Now here's a chance I'll never have again – to do some pre-history, and get to know about the earlier societies and the most *primitive* kinds of men."

When you meet as many people as I do, from different countries, different colours, different stages of social development with different drives, you become curious about what makes men tick, and what makes different men tick differently.

You wonder about the fundamental tension in a man, in mankind, between

19

body and soul. I got on to this at Gordonstoun and I grabbed the chance to follow it up a bit at Cambridge.

Charles ate the 30p dinner in hall, concluding:

Trinity has the worst food in Cambridge.

His social life at college:

It's a source of great regret to me that a lot of people are frightened of what other people would think of them if they came up and talked to me.

At one of the few parties I went to in the first year, I left early because they wouldn't put on the record-player as long as I was there.

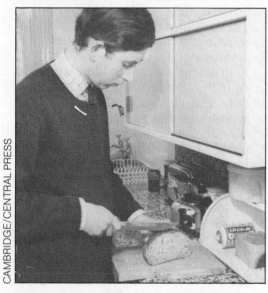

CAMBRIDGE/CENTRAL PRESS

The problems of fame and recognition:

I tried using disguise once at Cambridge because I wanted to go along and see what was happening in a demonstration. I borrowed an overcoat, put up the collar and pulled down a hat over my eyes. I just looked like me trying not to look like me! And everybody kept looking.

It's the same if you put on dark glasses: everyone wonders what on earth you're doing wearing dark glasses, particularly when the sun's not out! Even if you put on a false beard, or something, it'd blow away.

I often think that the whole fun of university life is breaking the rules...

Half the fun at Cambridge is to climb in at all hours of the night. It's a great challenge and it's been going on for years. What does it really matter?

But there are other things I agree with. The guest hours have been lengthened and you can have a girl or anybody else in your room until two o'clock in the morning instead of twelve o'clock. Well, that's all right.

Student Demonstrations:

I'm not the sort of person who might march or demonstrate, no. I don't agree with violence. I'm very suspicious of mobs and mob influence...

Some of those people who've demonstrated in Grosvenor Square never went with the intention of shouting or bashing a policeman on the head, but they were amazed when they found they did.

No, I'm not a demonstrating type, unless it came to the absolute crunch and I felt this was the only way of getting something done I felt strongly about.

I can't help feeling that, because students and many people feel so helpless and so anonymous in life and society, demonstrating is one useful way of making known your own particular opinions about world affairs, domestic matters and things like that.

It may also be because it's enjoyable, a lot of other people do it, it's the thing to do, it seems to be the thing to do.

I believe that a lot of people are very serious about it, but I can't help feeling that a lot of it is purely for the sake of change, and for the sake of doing something to change things, which from my point of view is pointless. You've got to do it constructively.

Aberystwyth.

In April 1969, Charles spent a term at the University College of Wales in Aberystwyth, learning Welsh before his investiture as Prince of Wales:

Misgivings had built up, but one had an exaggerated view of the situation.

I expect at Aberystwyth there may be one or two demonstrations, and as long as

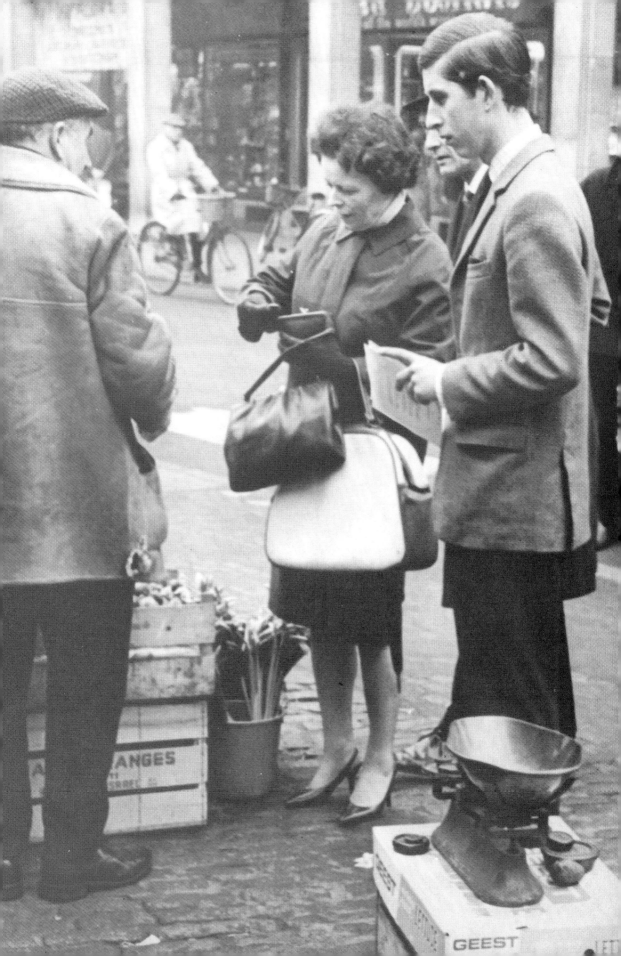

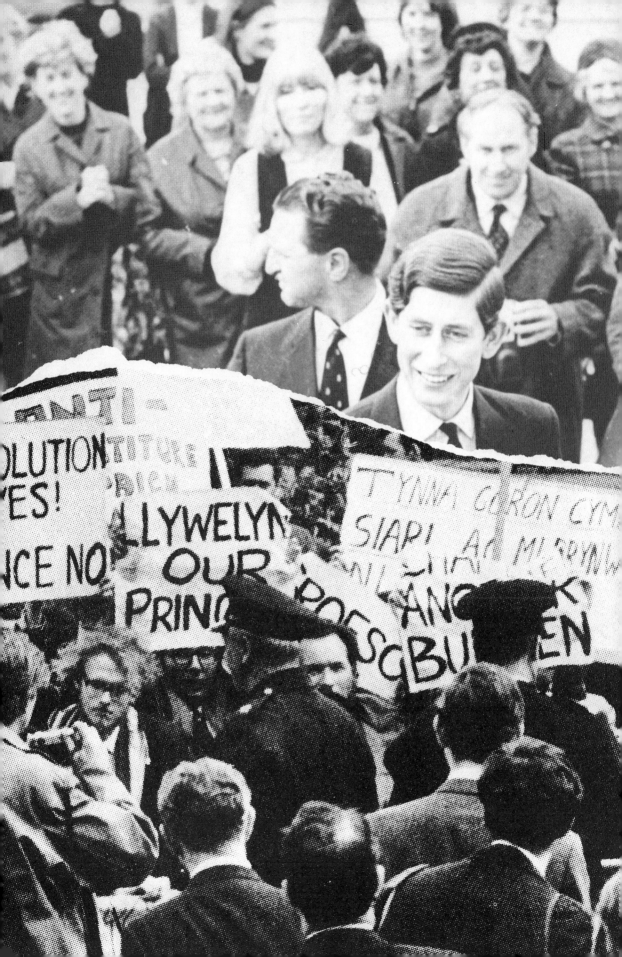

I don't get covered too much in egg and tomato, I'll be all right.

But I don't blame people demonstrating like that. They've never seen me before, they don't know what I'm like. I've hardly been to Wales and you can't really expect people to be over-zealous about having a so-called English Prince come amongst them.

I think once I've been there for eight weeks, things might improve!

I'm not an expert at heraldry and genealogy, but I'm told that I'm descended three times over from the original Welsh Princes. My grandmother, Queen Elizabeth, is descended twice over through both sides of her family, which is very interesting; and then I'm descended again on the other side. So I do have quite a lot of Welsh blood.

There was a Welsh Nationalist demonstration. Charles approached one of the demonstrators:

I had slight butterflies as I walked up, but I just went to see what it was these people were really getting at, you know? They were standing there and they were, I thought, perfectly ordinary people.

You somehow feel that, because they're demonstrating and they've got placards, they're a group apart – a sort of modern, ghastly phenomenon. Instead, I thought I might as well go and see.

So I asked one chap who was holding a placard what it was, what it meant, because it was in Welsh, and I'm afraid I haven't learnt it properly yet. So I asked him but he just hurled abuse at me, "Go home, Charlie," or something like that.

So, after I'd asked him more questions, I gave up. There was no point.

If I've learnt anything in the last eight weeks, it's been about Wales in particular, and its problems, and what these people feel about Wales. They're depressed about what might happen if they don't try to preserve the language and culture, which is unique and special to Wales. And if something is unique and special, I think it's well worth preserving.

I wouldn't have learned Welsh had I not been the Prince of Wales, but I couldn't

have worked at it as hard as I did if it hadn't been another entry into history, another way to find out about people, another way of satisfying human curiosity.

I like languages very much. I can never get very far with them, because I've never had enough time to pick up much of a vocabulary, or study the constructions. But I enjoy them. I've got a good ear, and I can mimic, and I like doing it.

I worked for eight weeks on my Welsh and it was damned hard – it's a hard language, very rich and very complex – but I enjoyed it. I spent an hour and a half with my Aberystwyth tutor the other day, and he was quite pleased with how much I'd remembered, and with my accent.

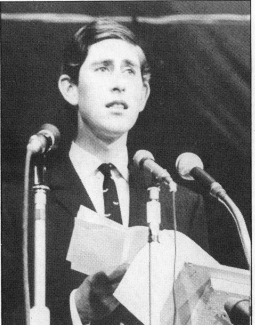

GIVING A WELSH SPEECH AT ABERYSTWYTH/PHOTO RAY DANIEL

I've learnt a lot about Welsh people – and about the way they operate in Aberystwyth. In fact, to live in a small town in Wales is rather interesting. And I wouldn't have been able to do it if I hadn't gone to university like this.

I've been most touched and amazed by the reaction of the people where I've been in Aberystwyth and the surrounding countryside, as to how they welcome me. I think it's shown me a lot about the way people live, which I wouldn't have found out otherwise, remaining in Cambridge…

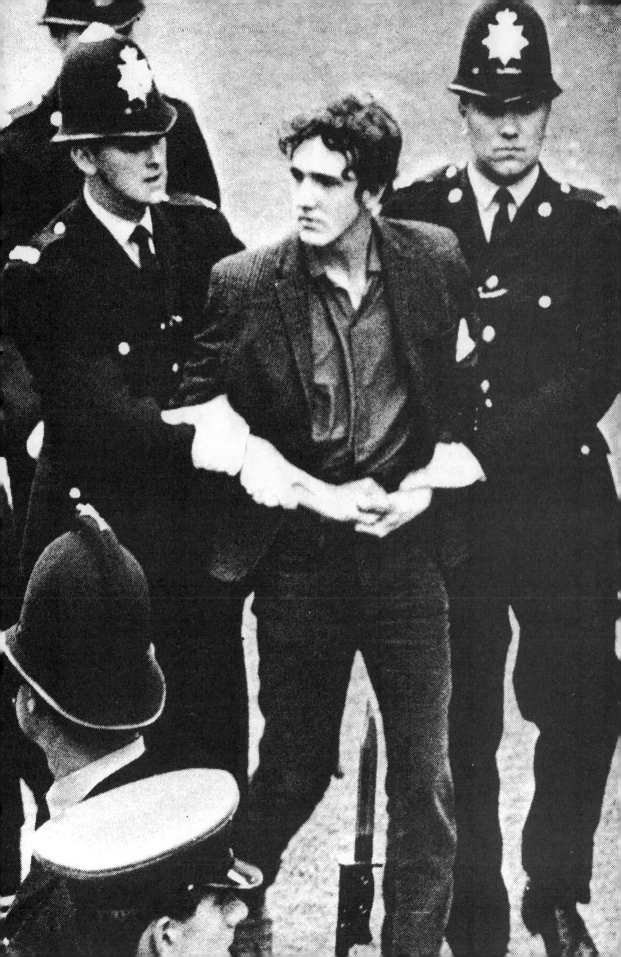

The Investiture.

Charles was created Prince of Wales during his time at Cheam. The announcement was made at the closing ceremony of the British & Commonwealth Games in July 1958:

I remember being acutely embarrassed when it was first announced. I heard this marvellous great cheer coming from the stadium in Cardiff, and I think for a little boy of nine it was rather bewildering. All the others turned and looked at me in amazement.

It perhaps didn't mean all that much then; later on, as I grew older, it became apparent what it meant.

Charles was formally invested as Prince of Wales at Caernarvon in July 1969:

During my investiture as Prince of Wales, I met so many people and waved so much that I woke up in the middle of the night waving my hand.

He was constantly on television at the time:

It's always me – I'm getting rather bored with my face.

Before the event:

It would be unnatural if I didn't feel any apprehension about it. I always wonder about what's going to happen in this sort of thing. But I think if I take this as it comes, it'll be much easier.

It'll be an exhausting day, but an enjoyable one, because I do enjoy ceremonies.

I don't really have the same sort of apprehension about it as the Duke of Windsor did. Perhaps one of the reasons is that I'm not as young as he was. He was only seventeen and, I think, felt very nervous and unsure of himself when he was at Dartmouth or somewhere.

He had a lot of friends of his own age, who, perhaps he felt, would take the mickey out of him because he was dressing up in pantaloons and things like that.

I don't feel so apprehensive. I'm not going to dress up as he did, and I'm older.

I look upon it, I think, as being a meaningful ceremony. I shall also be glad when it's over, because, having spent a year in the midst of controversy and talk between one side and another, it's become a friction point for many people.

Inevitably, when everybody is talking about an economic squeeze in the country, spending £250,000 on an apparently useless ceremony doesn't get

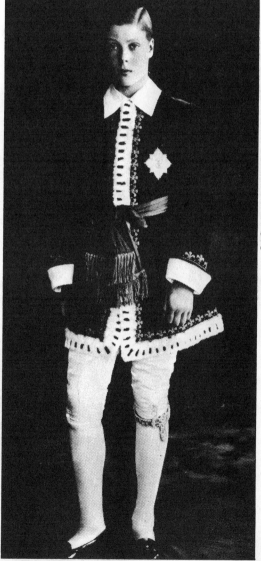

EDWARD AT HIS INVESTITURE/PHOTO POPPERFOTO

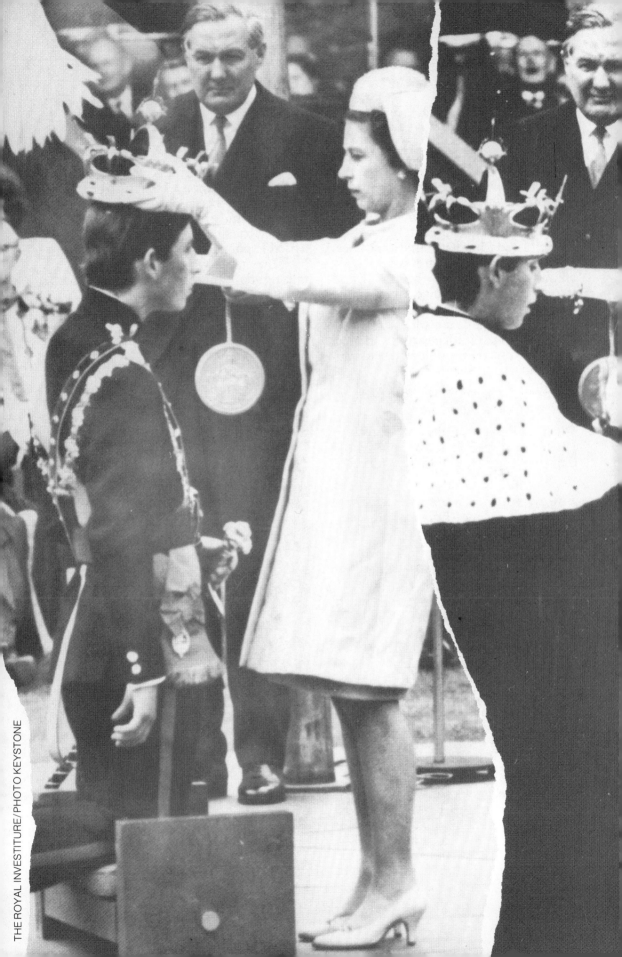

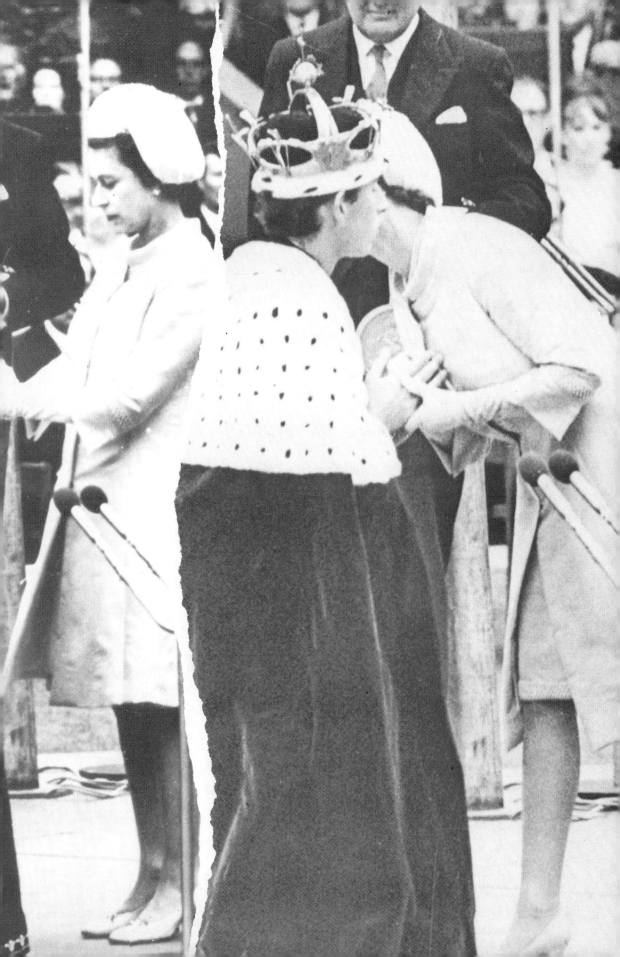

you positively anywhere, unless you think, "Oh well, we'll get some return in tourism, or investment from interested Americans."

My view of the situation is that, if you're going to have a ceremony like this, you should spend enough money to make it dignified, colourful, and worthy of Britain. But you shouldn't spend too much because it can just go on unnecessary things. On the other hand, you shouldn't spend too little because you make it skimped and you debase the whole object of the exercise.

Anybody looking at it from the outside, would wonder why on earth we went to all the bother of having a ceremony like this in an open castle, part ruin, in which there is hardly any room. If it rains we all get wet, and the Household Cavalry are having to stay in tents, in people's gardens and parks. The soldiers have to be billeted everywhere.

There is only one road and one railway into the town and the Royal train will take up the one line. I can see all the rest of the special trains will be backed-up to London!

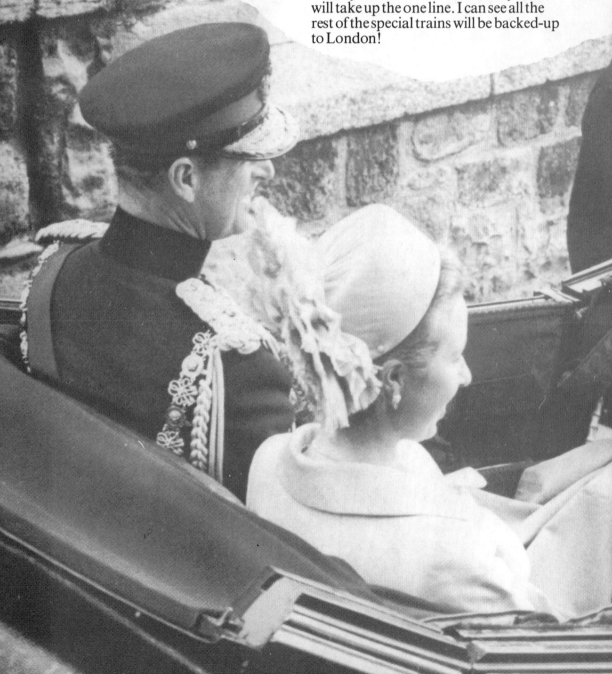

The Investiture.

PHOTO CENTRAL PRESS

At the ceremony the Queen and Charles exchanged the kiss of fealty:

I, Charles, Prince of Wales, do become your liege man of life and limb and of earthly worship, and faith and truth I will bear unto you to live and die against all manner of folks.

Speaking in Welsh, Charles went on to say:

The demands of a Prince of Wales have altered, but I am determined to serve and to try as best I can to live up to those demands, whatever they might be, in the rather uncertain future.

One thing I am clear about is that Wales needs to look forward without forsaking the traditions and essential aspects of her past. The past can be just as much a stimulus to the future as anything else. By the affirmation of your loyalty today, for which I express my gratitude, this will not simply be a faint hope.

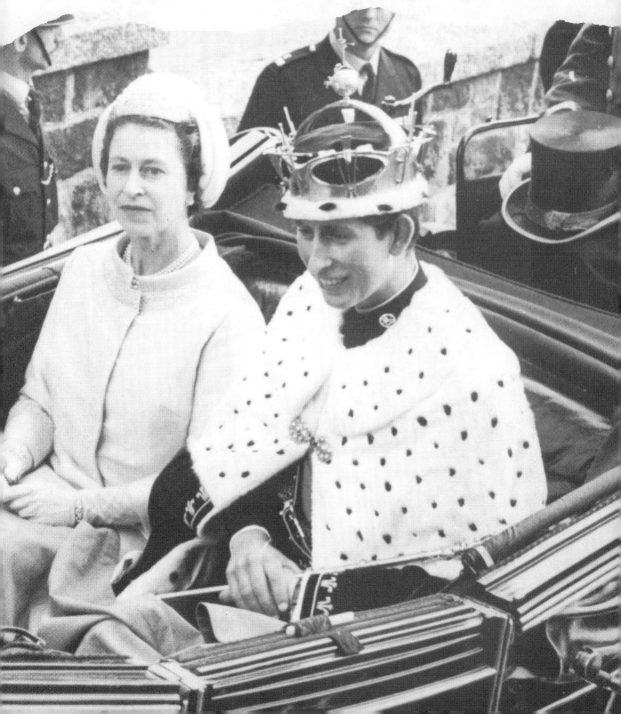

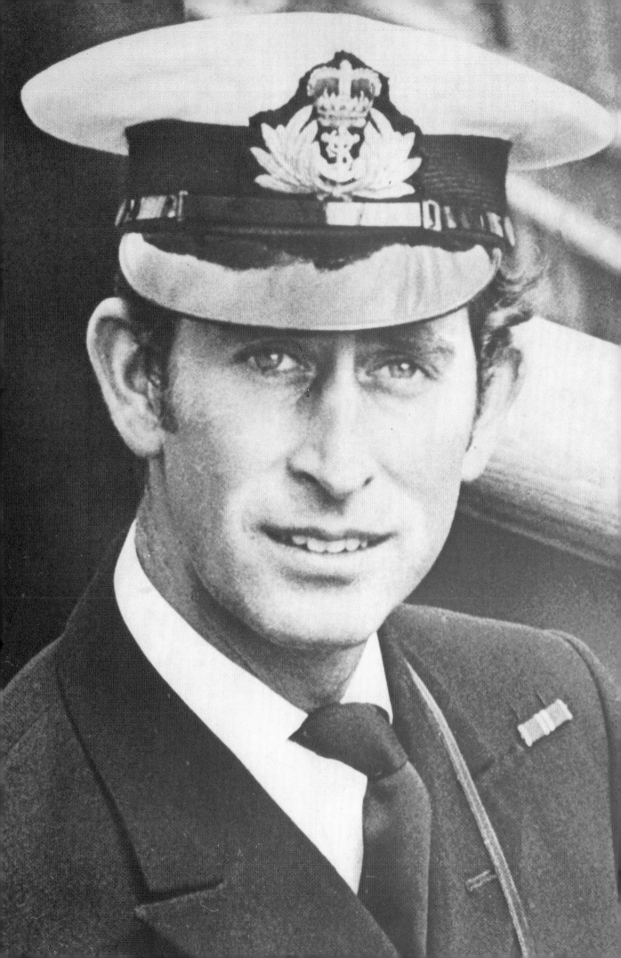

The Services.

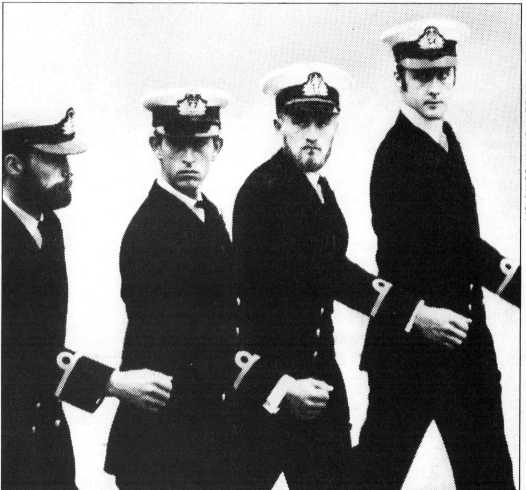

PASSING OUT PARADE AT DARTMOUTH, 1971

I'm going to be a sailor – so long as my parents will let me. (Age 11)

His plans for a career in the Royal Navy were announced while he was still at Cambridge:

I'm looking forward to it very much. I hope I shall not be too seasick.

After six months of RAF training, Charles joined the Navy in September 1971:

A period in the Services gives you great experience and responsibility: of life, of discipline, and, above all, of people and how to deal with people. To discipline them and to be disciplined by them.

It's pointless and ill-informed to say that I'm entering a profession trained in killing.

In the first place, the Services are there for fast, efficient and well-trained action in defence. Surely the Services must attract a large number of duty-conscious people? Otherwise, who else would subject themselves to being square-bashed, shouted at by petty officers and made to do ghastly things in force ten gales?

I'm entering the RAF and then the Navy because I believe I can contribute something to this country by so doing. To

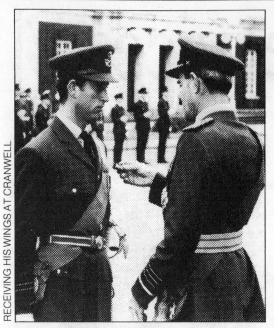

RECEIVING HIS WINGS AT CRANWELL

me, it's a worthwhile occupation and one which I'm convinced will stand me in good stead for the rest of my life.

I feel that if one is going to get involved in the whole spectrum of life in this country,

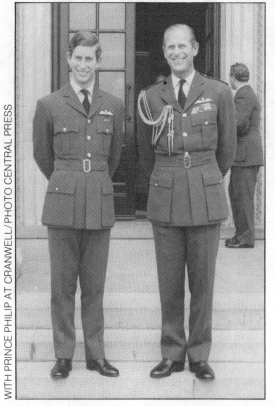

WITH PRINCE PHILIP AT CRANWELL / PHOTO CENTRAL PRESS

then one should get to know about the Services. One should get to know about the Navy particularly because, ultimately, our security and everything depends upon the Navy. It always has done throughout history and always will.

I tried very hard to be as professional as possible. I hope I demonstrated a reasonable amount of enthusiasm. The difficulty was that I'd done a shortened course of introduction to the Navy and a fairly short period of training. I therefore had to try that little bit harder to assimilate the vast amount of technical information and all the navigational problems rather more quickly than other people had to do.

The trouble is that people expect me to be a genius at the very least, and to achieve the impossible rather sooner than in the immediate. I think I eventually managed to accustom myself to the pace and made people realise I couldn't necessarily live up to the programme they had mapped out.

But I think the Navy meant a great deal to me because I was basically brought up in it. My father was in it; my grandfather; my great-uncle, Lord Mountbatten; and my great-grandfathers, Prince Louis of Battenberg and King George V.

I had a very glamorous, romantic idea about it, which wasn't always borne out because there are an awful lot of mundane tasks to be carried out. But I also think the Navy's history, and the fact that it has saved this country from disaster on more than one occasion, gave me a particular interest in it, as something somebody in my position ought to know a reasonable amount about.

I hope that people in the Navy feel that I've taken an interest and can sympathise with their difficulties and aspirations.

I think it's very important that I should understand something about the defence of my country. I think the Navy ought to mean a great deal to this country – this island.

Then there is the educational value of the Services. If you want to understand what they've done for me, you can see what

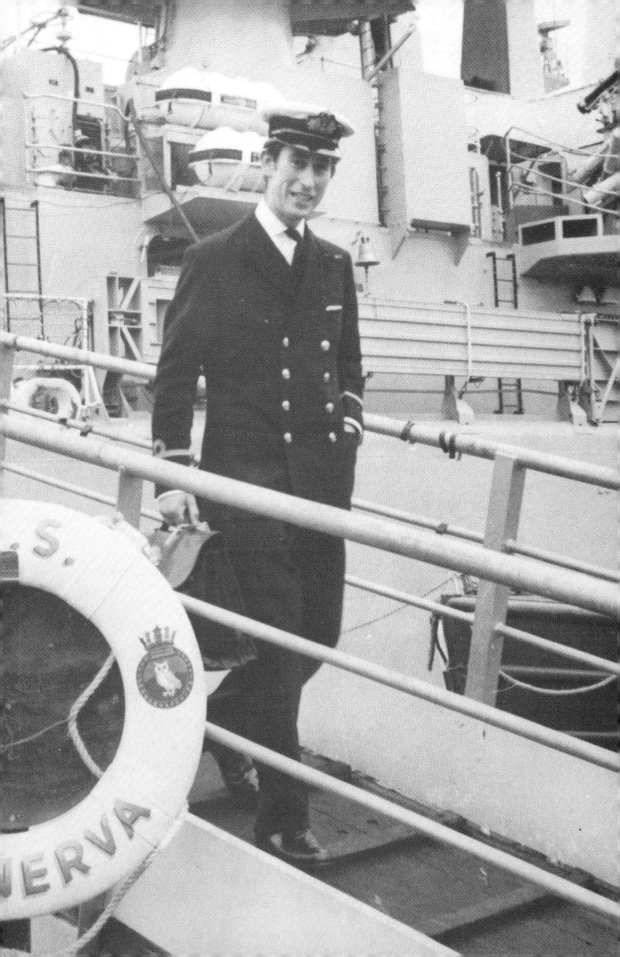

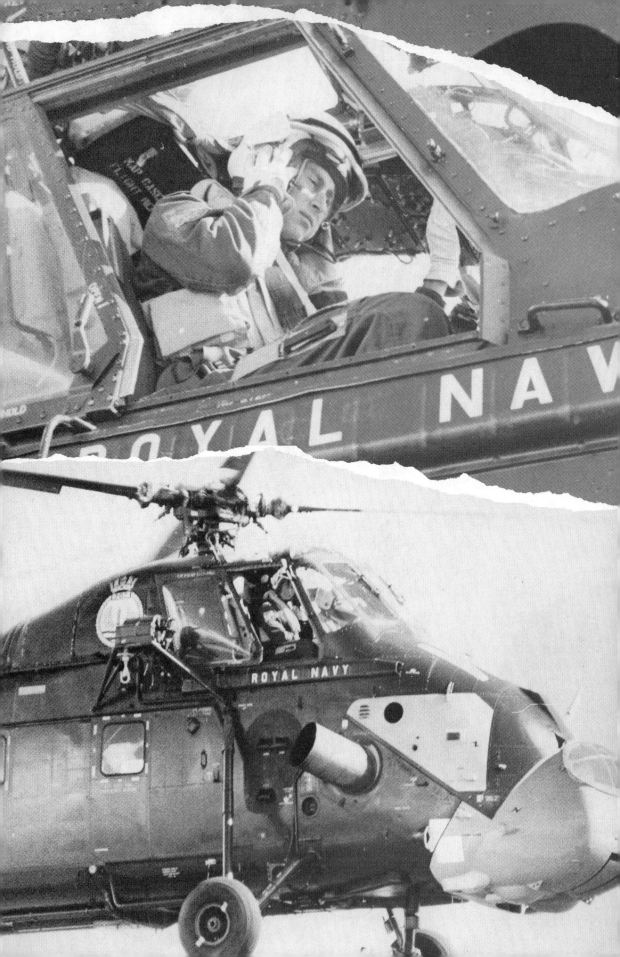

they've done for thousands of other young men from every walk of life.

With the RAF of course, there was the particular bonus of flying. You have responsibilities to and for other human beings in all three Services, but most – I found, anyway – in the Navy. You're all together out there, at sea, in that small community, cut off. It's a very intense communal life.

Flying.

While in the Navy, Charles learned to fly helicopters:

I adore flying and I personally cannot think of a better combination than Navy flying – being at sea and being able to fly at the same time. I found it very exciting, very rewarding and very stimulating – also bloody terrifying, sometimes.

I think people who fly in the Fleet Air Arm are a very special breed, particularly those chaps who fly Buccaneers and Phantoms. They are taking all kinds of risks; taking off from and landing on carriers, particularly at night, is no joke.

If you're living dangerously, it tends to make you appreciate life that much more and to want to live it to the fullest. Fleet Air Arm flyers are some of the most invigorating and amusing people I've come across. I enjoyed every minute of the helicopter course at Yeovilton.

In the Queen's Flight, you tend to take off in a helicopter or aeroplane, fly in a straight line, land, get out and shake hands with a lot of people.

But at Yeovilton one did all sorts of things – commando flying, rocket firing, and landing on carriers and the back-end of ships in howling gales. I found the course easier, and got the knack more quickly than I had expected.

Many people forget that a helicopter is an inherently unstable machine. With a helicopter, you've got to expect something to go wrong any minute and be ready to do something about it pretty quickly, because if you don't, you drop like a stone. If you do make a mistake, your life often depends on taking the correct action immediately.

It's very challenging. There's that superb mixture of fear and enjoyment which comes over me.

It's marvellous when things are going right and you can pick up a reference on the ground and not bother with the map. Then that panic when you don't really know where you are and you've got to sort it out yourself. It's so exciting.

I've given myself a fright or two. The other day, we were going along quite well

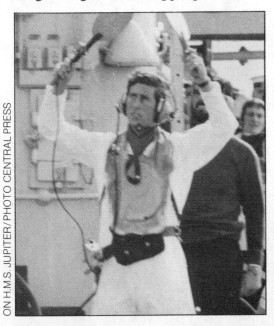

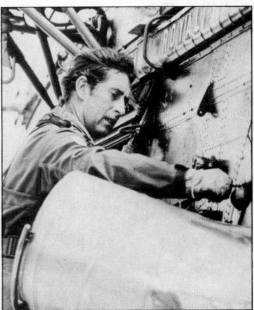

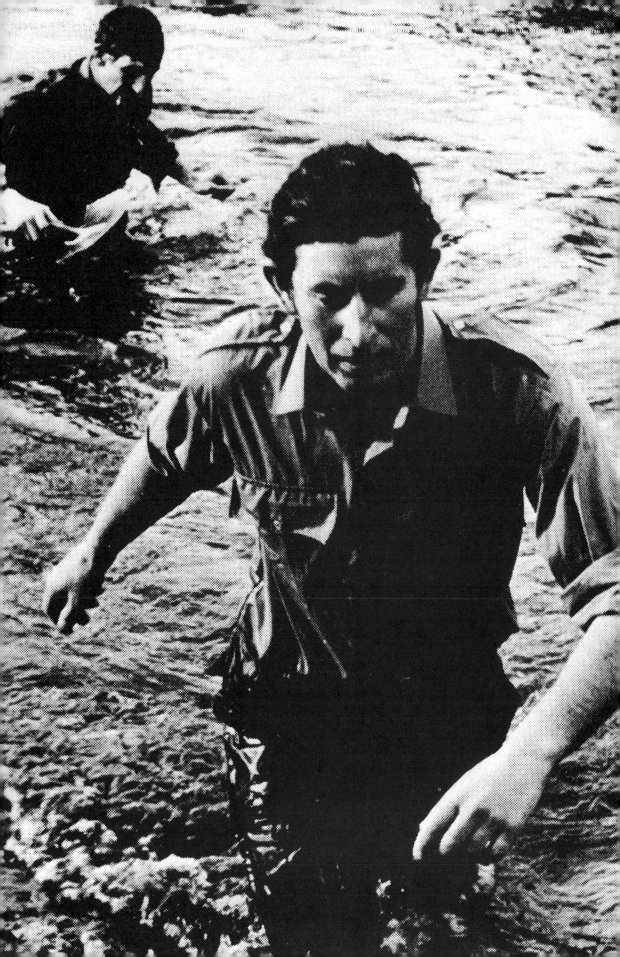

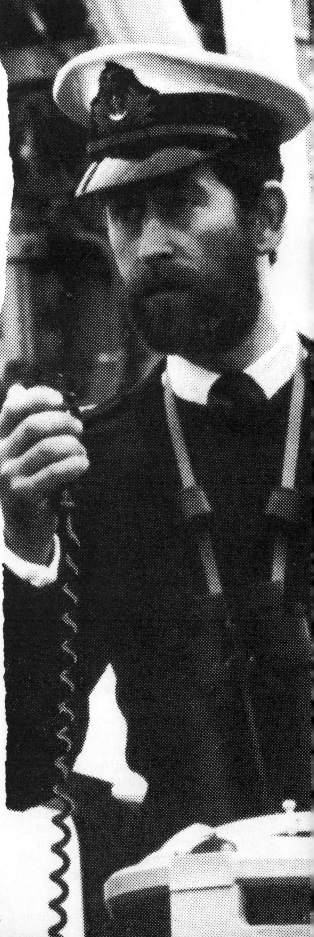

when flames suddenly started to shoot out of the engine on my side, making extraordinary "whoof-whoof" noises. All the instruments were twitching away.

Fortunately, I was with the senior pilot of the squadron so we shut down the engine and landed in a ploughed field beside a motorway – much to everybody's amazement!

Part of our duties as helicopter pilots involves carrying Royal Marines. It's considered a good idea for the pilots to find out what the Marines have to put up with, from first-hand knowledge.

So I went down to do the Marines assault course at Lympstone in Devon, to do what the Marines charmingly call a "Tarzan" course – a most horrifying expedition where you have to swing over small chasms, slide down ropes at death-defying speeds and then walk across wires and up rope ladders strung between a pole and a tree. All sorts of ghastly things.

Anyway, I survived that and came out with my knees trembling in fear and trepidation. Then we had to do a form of survival course which involved crawling through tunnels half-filled with water, then running across the moor and back.

The technical side of flying was a bit of a problem:

From the flying point of view, my arithmetic is not as fast as some other peoples.

Maths taken in its pure context is misery, I think. I find it boring. I'm one of those people who prefers ideas rather than numbers. I could never understand maths. I always thought it was the way I'd been taught originally that made me so hopeless, but, on the other hand, perhaps I just don't have a mathematical mind.

HMS Bronington.

In February, 1976, Charles was given his own naval command – the mine-sweeper HMS Bronington:

It's given me a marvellous opportunity to get as close to the "ordinary" British chap as possible.

After his appointment, he told a meeting of the Grand Order of Water Rats:

If any of you are considering sailing in the North Sea next year, or if you

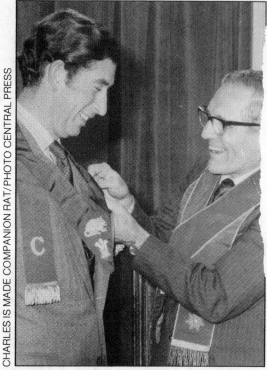

CHARLES IS MADE COMPANION RAT/PHOTO CENTRAL PRESS

happen to own an oil rig in Scottish waters, I strongly advise you to increase your insurance contributions forthwith.

On being in a position of command:

One of the most important things is to be as honest and as genuine as possible. People can always see through you if you're being artificial – particularly a sailor.

And you've got to have a sense of humour, because half the battle is giving as good as you get, accepting the teasing and the ribbing.

But the most important thing about a position of responsibility or command is to get a chap to do something willingly. I know they'll moan and groan. But having done it they'll say, "That wasn't too bad, sir, was it?"

I often think there are two types of leadership. One for the more aggressive, dominant person who imposes his will forcibly on people and gains their respect through his sheer determination and

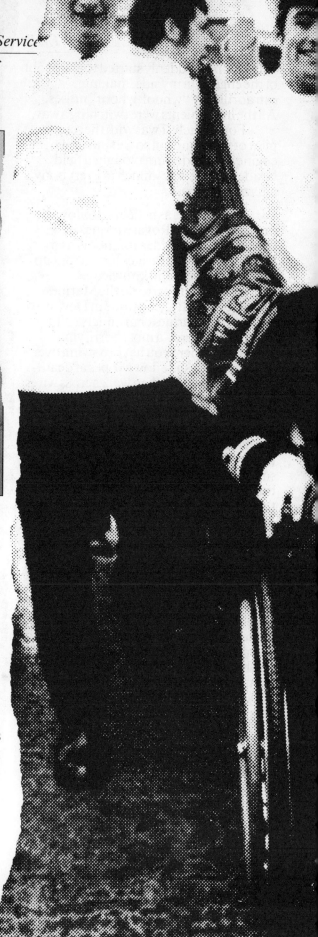

LEAVING H.M.S. BRONINGTON/PHOTO PRESS ASSOCIATION

ability. The other is someone who tends to charm people and is more friendly. People feel it's worth doing something for him because they like the person.

In the summer of 1976, Charles organised a family day aboard. The invitation read:

It is hoped the trip will give a clearer idea of life at sea than can normally be extracted from your exhausted menfolk when they return home.

Charles.

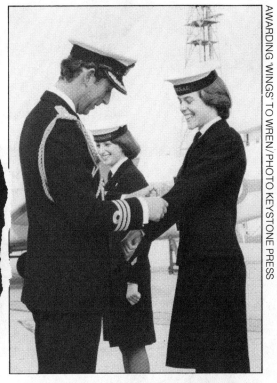

AWARDING 'WINGS' TO WREN / PHOTO KEYSTONE PRESS

When nineteen-year-old Jane Chapman, Miss Spotlight of Rosyth Naval Base, came aboard, Charles welcomed her:

I presume you've taken the pill this morning. Of course, I mean the seasick pill.

HMS Bronington was the only ship in the Navy ever to make Charles seasick. He said of his first ten weeks at sea:

They took ten years off my life . . . I feel about eighty.

Charles left the Navy in December, 1976:

There are other things to do and it would be rather selfish of me if I remained locked away here. It has been great fun, a splendid experience.

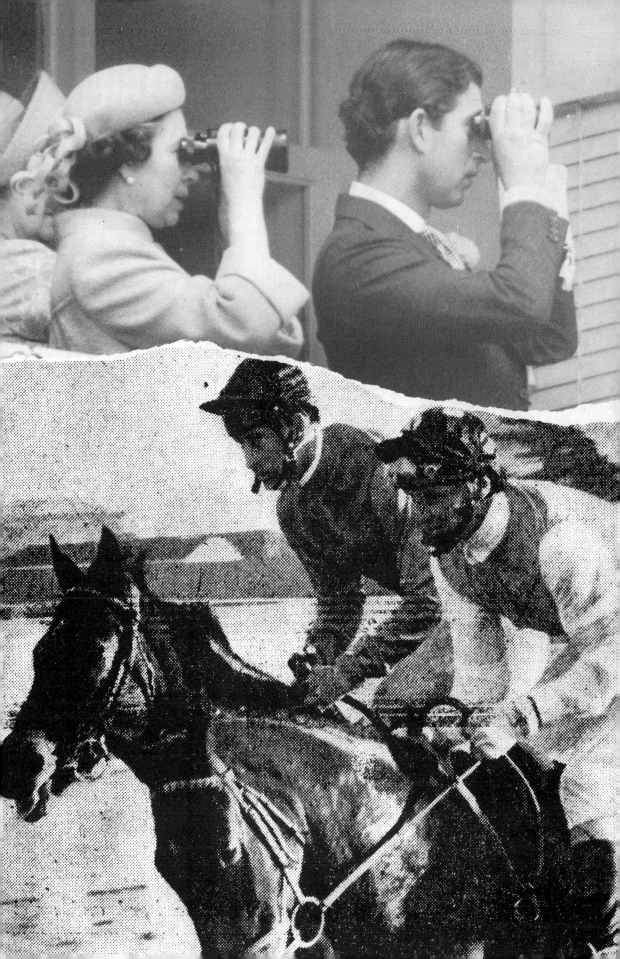

Sport.

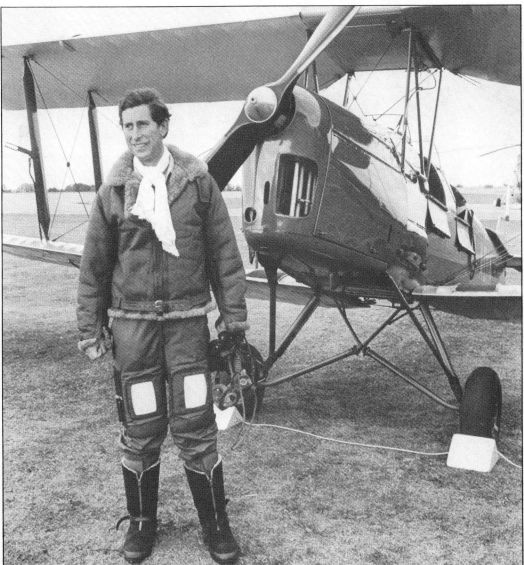

PHOTO CENTRAL PRESS

I believe in living life dangerously and I think a lot of others do too.

I am a hopeless individual because I happen to enjoy an element of adventure and danger. I think that if you occasionally live dangerously it helps you appreciate life. Not only that, you discover your own abilities which, perhaps, you did not know were there.

I'm stupid enough to like trying things. I like to see if I can challenge myself to do something that is potentially hazardous, just to see if mentally I can accept that challenge and carry it out.

I like to try all sorts of things because they appeal to me. I'm one of those people who doesn't like sitting and watching someone else doing something. I don't like going to

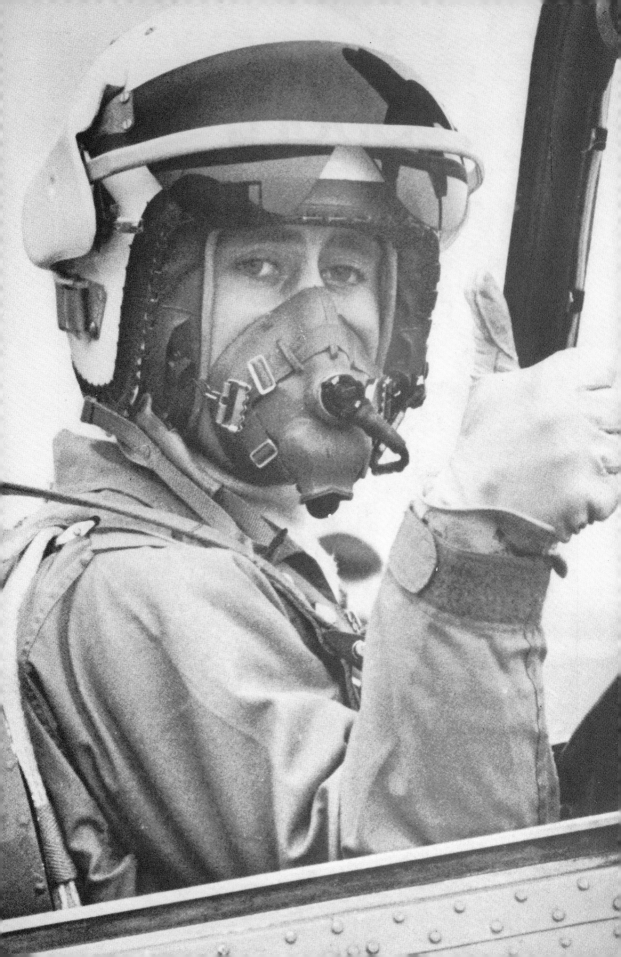

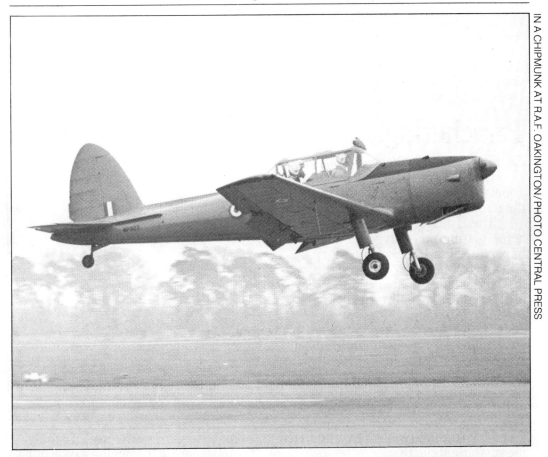

IN A CHIPMUNK AT R.A.F. OAKINGTON/PHOTO CENTRAL PRESS

the races to watch horses thundering up and down – I'd rather be riding one myself.

Flying.

Charles made his first solo flight in January 1969:

It's imprinted on my mind indelibly. I suppose I worried about it for a bit ... the thought of actually having to go solo and whether I was capable of doing it. Whether I'd remember the right things to do.

I always thought I was going to be terrified. I was dreading the moment throughout training when I'd have to go up alone. But on the day I went solo, the instructor taxied up to the end of the runway, suddenly climbed out and said, "You're on your own, mate!"

So, there I was, and I hardly had time to get butterflies in my tummy before taking off.

I was wondering whether I could do it, but the moment I was in the air it was absolutely marvellous. There was no instructor to breathe down my neck and the aeroplane flew much better because he had gone and the weight was not there.

I had a wonderful time. I flew round and round and admired the scenery. I controlled my butterflies. Then I did a perfect landing – as it turned out, I never did a better one after that.

That had been the only thing worrying me during the flight. I had visions of going around and around until eventually the fuel ran out. But all was well.

Charles described his approach to flying:

It's a mixture between fear and supreme enjoyment. I'd like to go on flying for as long as I could but, once out of the Navy, the only flying I could do would be from one engagement to another.

I like trying my hand at things and if people say, "Do you want to have a go?", I usually say, "Yes."

He returned to Cranwell in February 1977, to brush up his flying and aerobatics:

I've forgotten so much – especially those convolutions of the stomach when you go into a roll or a loop. Dangerous? No, it's more dangerous crossing the road.

Parachuting.

Charles described his first parachute jump:

I purposely didn't think very much about the whole operation until I got into the aeroplane.

Then I did get slightly apprehensive before getting out – they say you should have butterflies. It makes you sharp, I discovered, because out I went the instant this hairy flight sergeant shouted in my ear and gave me a tap on the shoulder.

The slip-stream is terrific, particularly getting out of the side of an Andover. You appear to be flipped on your back. The next thing I knew, my feet were above my head . . . which was very odd. Either I've got hollow legs or something, it doesn't often happen. The first thing I thought was, "They didn't tell me anything about this."

The next thing I knew, my legs were tangled in the rigging lines, so I was looking up at them and coming down in a

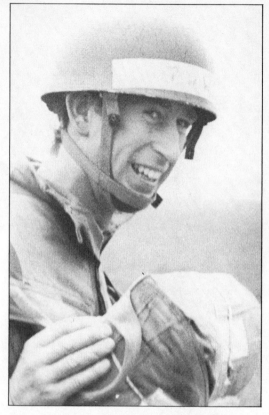

sort of U-shape. I said to myself calmly, "Your legs are in the rigging so you must remove them." So I removed them – fortunately by about 800 feet. Then I had a lovely sail down to sea level.

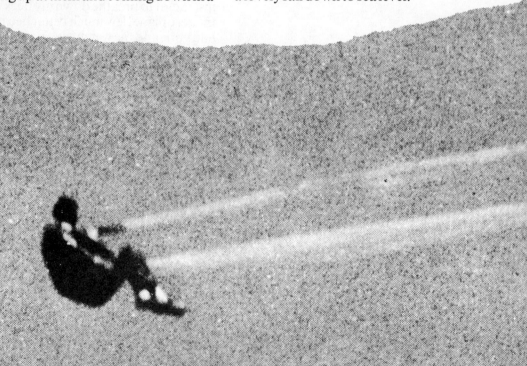

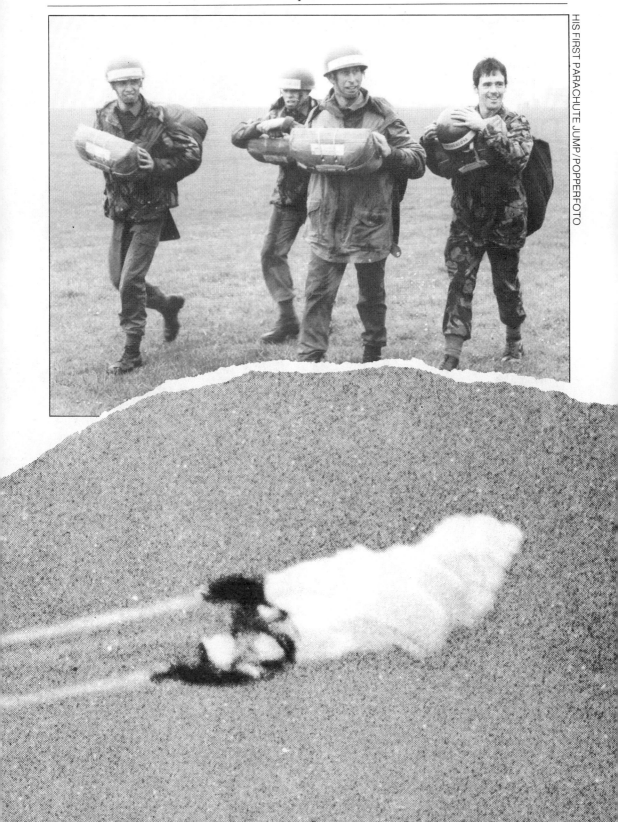

Of course, I forgot to inflate my life jacket because I'd enjoyed it so much. But the Royal Marines were roaring around in little rubber boats underneath and I was out of the water within ten seconds.

Diving.

Charles explored a wreck off the Virgin Islands:

There is a supreme satisfaction in life below the waves, experiencing the extraordinary sensation of swimming inside the hull of an old schooner as if it

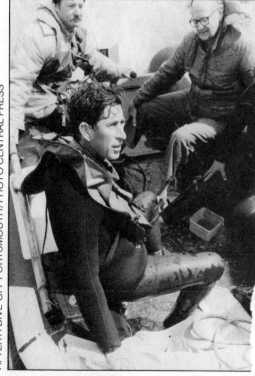

AFTER A DIVE OFF PORTSMOUTH / PHOTO CENTRAL PRESS

THE ARCTIC / PHOTO ANWAR HUSSEIN

were some vast green cathedral filled with shoals of fish.

I can well imagine the disease which grips divers and dedicates them to their hobby or profession.

Charles dived in Arctic waters from HMS Hermes and walked upside down on a fathom of ice:

I lowered myself gingerly into the water, which by now was covered with newly formed pieces of ice – rather like Crème de menthe frappé – and sank like a

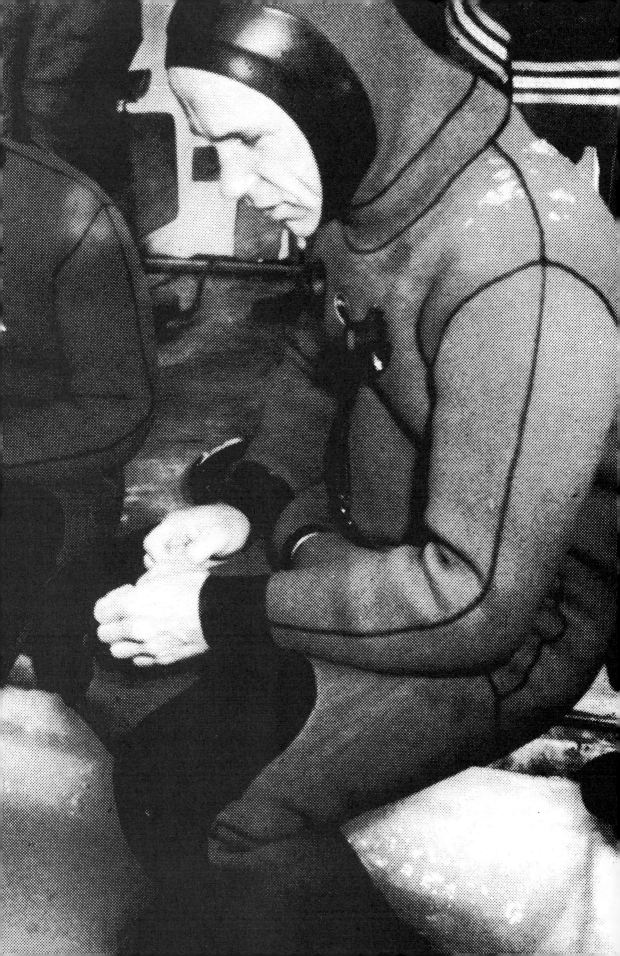

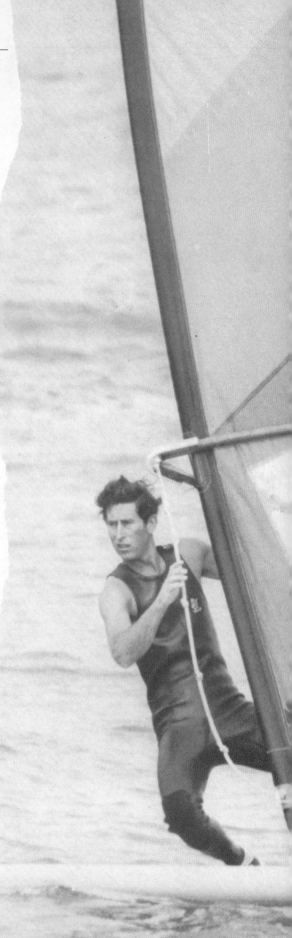

great orange walrus into the ice-covered world below.

Once at the bottom of the six-foot shaft, the similarity with a walrus vanished abruptly to be replaced by a resemblance to a dirigible balloon underwater. I found it extremely hard to preserve my balance and had to struggle to stay upright.

Despite the rubber hood, the water felt decidedly cold around my mouth and a few other edges, not to mention the fact that, with heavy gloves on my hands, I couldn't get my fingers onto my mask in order to clear my ears. So I "ballasted" myself out at a depth which was not too painful and took stock of the situation.

It was a fascinating, eerie world of greyish-greenish light that met my gaze and above all was the roof of ice which disappeared into the distance.

The visibility was extraordinarily good. The water was virtually silt-free due to the lack of wave action – the ambient light visibility was 100 feet.

I couldn't resist giving it a try! The result of my upside-down walk was highly comical in the extreme. I only partly succeeded.

What was fascinating was to see the exhaust bubbles trapped on the underside of the ice, spread out like great pools of shimmering mercury.

The icicles looked like beautiful, transparent wafers. Nestling in the gaps between the wafers were lots of shrimp-like creatures.

Other Sports.

Golf:
    The game does not amuse me.

Skateboarding:
    Had I known I'd have the chance to try a skateboard, I would, of course, have brought my helmet with me…

Rugger:
    They always put me in the second row, the worst place in the scrum.

Surfing:
    I've joined the surf club (in Wales) which is rather fun. I try to surf as often as I

can. It's a marvellous form of exercise, and you feel twice as well afterwards as before.

Ski-ing:
　　We British must ski on.

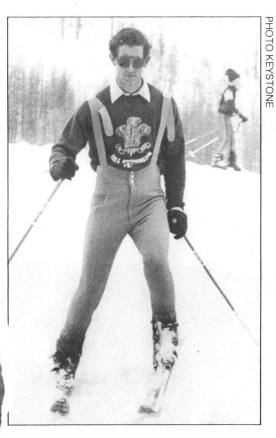

PHOTO KEYSTONE

Rock Climbing:
　　I don't particularly like the idea of having to cling to a rock face by the fingernails.

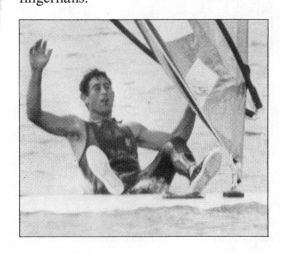

Polo:

I love the game, I love the ponies, I love the exercise. It's the one team game I can play. It's also a very convenient game for me as long as I spend my weekends at Windsor.

It isn't convenient to play football; you can't just nip out of Windsor Castle and enjoy a soccer game.

But if I knew that there was immense criticism of my playing polo, I'd have to think about it. You can't have everything you want, even if you feel it does no harm. People's susceptibilities count.

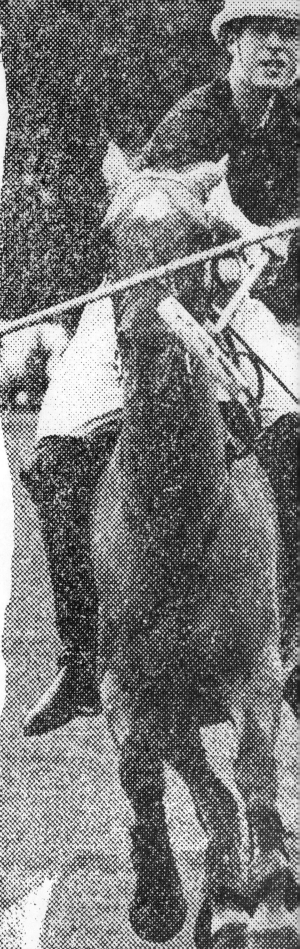

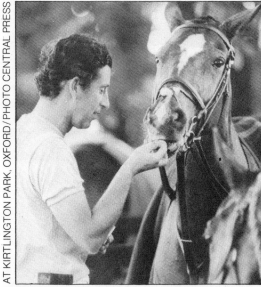

AT KIRTLINGTON PARK, OXFORD/ PHOTO CENTRAL PRESS

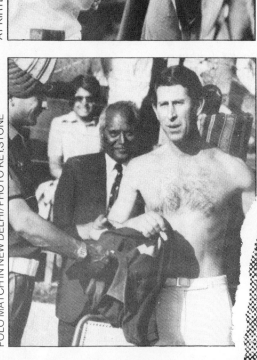

POLO MATCH IN NEW DELHI/ PHOTO KEYSTONE

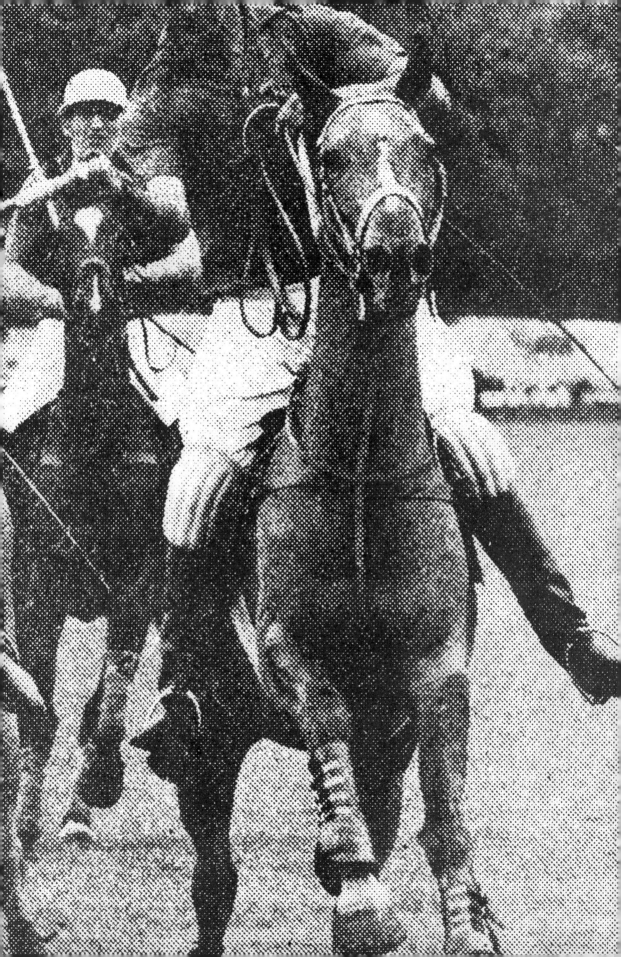

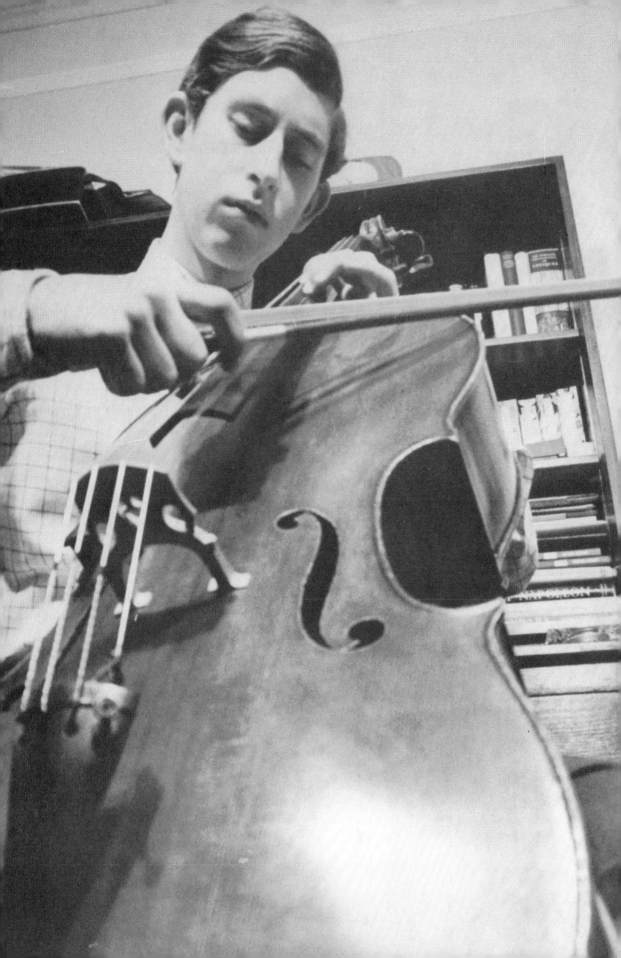

Hobbies.

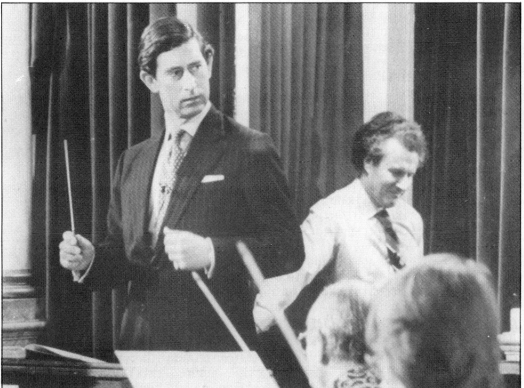

CONDUCTING MOZART'S 'THE MAGIC FLUTE'/PHOTO CENTRAL PRESS

Music.

I find that music moves me very deeply. A beautiful picture, or being out on a mountain with the wind and the trees – I feel very deeply about that sort of thing.

I like music very much. I liked playing it – I haven't so much time now – and I like listening to it. The trouble is, though you haven't much time for listening, you have even less time for practising, and if you don't practise you simply can't enjoy your own noise.

When I went to prep school, I learned the piano: no good. Then I took up the trumpet. I rather enjoyed it, but one of the music teachers – who happened to be German – didn't: she couldn't stand the noise.

I used to play the trumpet in the school orchestra. We made such an awful noise, in the back row. I can hear the music teacher now. We'd all be playing away and making a hell of a din, when suddenly, she couldn't stand it any longer. She'd put down her violin, we'd all stop, and she'd shout – she had a heavy German accent and somehow, that made her sound more agonised – "Ach! Zoze trumpetz! Ach! Zoze trumpetz! Stawp Zoze Trumpetz." So I gave up the trumpet.

Later, I began to think about the 'cello. It had such a rich, deep sound. One night, I was at the Festival Hall and I heard Jacqueline Du Pré playing with her husband Daniel Barenboim. I'd never heard sounds like it. I said, "I must try this." So I did. I couldn't keep it up. I remember playing in a performance of Beethoven's Fifth one night. It was a wonderful experience, but I couldn't play concentratedly enough to avoid being confused.

Pop music I enjoy as it comes. I don't go out of my way to listen to pop sessions, but if it's there – if I happen to catch it – I enjoy it.

Whom do I like? Well, it's a bit unfair on others, because I can't always bring a name to mind when asked – particularly since I listen at random, not selectively. I like The Seekers. The Beatles sang splendid music – and wrote great music.

Jazz I enjoy. But I'm no connoisseur. But I really prefer classical music, because I find the more I listen to classical works, the more I get out of them. Pop music may pall after two or three hearings. The Beatles were an exception for me: the more I heard them, the more I enjoyed them.

In classical music my taste, such as it is, is conservative: Bach, Mozart and Beethoven. But there are exceptions, such as Berlioz.

Once, I was listening to Richard Baker's 'These You Have Loved,' on the BBC. He played a piece by Berlioz from a choral work I'd never heard of: 'L'enfance du Christ.' I thought, "I must get it." I play it now, often. There's a certain passage in it which is so moving I'm reduced to tears every time.

I'm not mad keen on much modern music. I love *tunes,* and I love *rhythm.* Rhythm is deep in me – if I hear rhythmic music I just want to get up and dance. That's one of the reasons why I had such a marvellous time in the West Indies.

A good deal of modern music is tuneless, as far as I'm concerned. But it can grow on you with familiarity. For instance, once I sang in Benjamin Britten's *Saint Nicholas,* and I didn't appreciate it at all at first. After several rehearsals, I began to enjoy it.

The same tended to be true with the *Dream of Gerontius,* in which I also sang while at school and in the choir. I now become intensely moved by listening to it.

Have you ever sung in a big choir? It's marvellous. I sang in the Bach 'B Minor Mass' – there's nothing like it. I don't know whether it's the volume of the voices, or the sense of participation – you're not just listening, you're helping to make the sound – but it's really very exciting.

But it's something you can enjoy only if you keep at it. You can't just turn up and say, "I like singing in choirs. Can I sing in yours tonight, please?"

One of the things I really enjoy about being Patron of the Royal Opera is having the chance to see as many operas as I can and to find out more about it.

I like to think I can go whenever I want to, at short notice – turfing people out of the Royal Box so I can get a seat!

Painting.

I'm one of those people who leaps from one thing to another. I took up water-colour painting about two years ago. It's frightfully difficult. I tried to get some lessons from Edward Seago who was a great Norfolk painter. He died, sadly, last year. He'd never given lessons in his life. He said, "All right. I'll give you a lesson, but only one."

I just sat and watched in awe as he proceeded to paint a picture entirely from memory. Before you could say "knife," in fifteen minutes, there was this marvellous little picture of two Thames barges. I said, "Can I have it?" and he said, "Of course."

I'm going to take more lessons. It's very rewarding, very hard work. And marvellous for Christmas presents!

Theatre.

I enjoy very much going to the theatre and to concerts when I can. The quality of plays and the music is astonishingly good. I do think London has extremely high standards and is one of the great cultural centres of the world, one of the great theatrical centres.

Of course, one could easily say that one's own country has the best of everything. But I think in this case it's probably true.

I love, as I say, going to the theatre because I rather enjoy acting and therefore I like live entertainment.

I enjoy films as well. But there's a special atmosphere to the theatre. I like going out

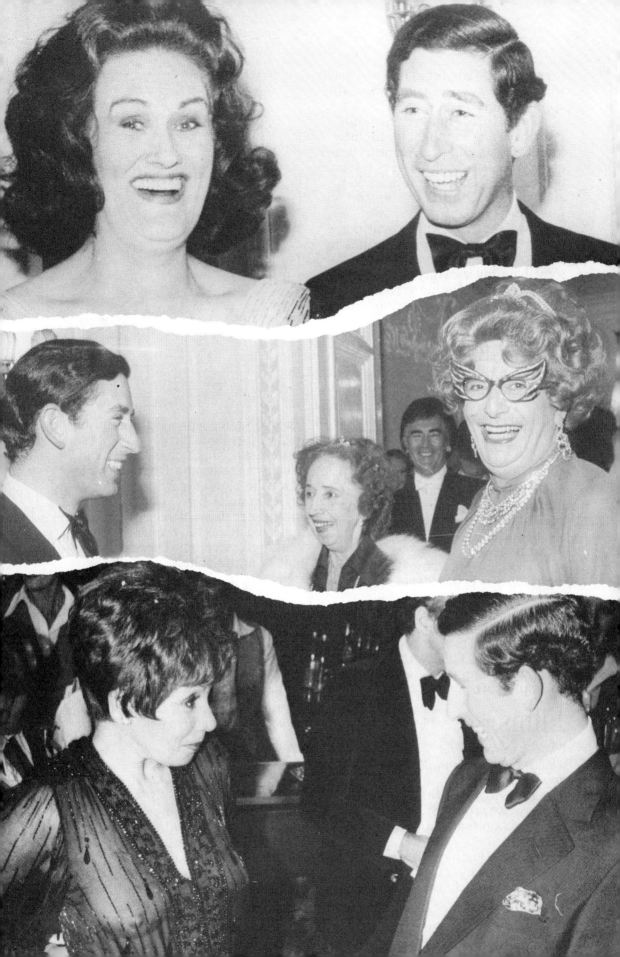

to enjoy a good laugh, but I have to watch who I take because their name inevitably appears in the papers!

I went to see a thing called *Absurd Person Singular*. I thought it extremely funny; very slick and fast. I'd never heard of Mr. Alan Ayckbourn. I hadn't seen any of his plays before. I believe he's also got another one on, called *The Norman Conquests*.

I was sad to see, when I went, that there were very few people in the theatre. I suppose it was the wrong night or something, but it was my birthday, and I thought it would be fun to take the Queen and Princess Alexandra out to the theatre.

Television.

Very much a question of time. It's weeks since I had a night on my own. I've had some very interesting evenings in and out of the Palace in the past few weeks, but not one when I could say to myself, "I'll have a look at a TV programme."

When I do get a chance, I love watching selected things. But I find television a great drug and, before you know where you are, you just sit there with your eyes becoming square and everybody saying, "Oh, come on, we'll watch it a bit longer."

There are some things I love watching like Monty Python, The Goodies, or certain documentaries.

The other night there was a programme on how birds navigate thousands of miles across oceans. It was most intriguing. Those sort of programmes are marvellous, but there's an awful lot of tripe.

Films.

Charles saw an X-film, 'Percy's Progress,' while staying in Cornwall, causing much press comment:

It was frightfully funny. There were about twelve people in the cinema – two courting couples and some other curious characters.

I think it just happened because we were in the Duchy of Cornwall area; that added to the chances of publicity.

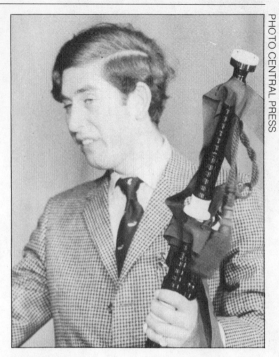

Everybody recognised me instantly in the pubs. Marvellous old boys in caps came up and said, "Like ter shake yer hand." They were charming. One old boy produced his Home Guard certificate, signed by my grandfather.

But that sort of thing never gets reported. It's all this business about looking for scrumpy. Everybody must think I'm an alcoholic.

I mean, I don't go to these things for serious reasons. At the time of the Okehampton incident, we were on an exercise in the middle of Dartmoor. The tent was sopping wet and everybody decided to go off. What would have been the point of my being stand-offish and saying, "I'm not going to the pub, I'm not going to the cinema." As it happens, it wasn't even a blue movie.

Acting.

Charles made his acting début while at Cambridge:

I spent many hours with a tape recorder listening to a long soliloquy of Richard Hunchback spoken by Sir Laurence before taking this on myself.

I must have been either incredibly good or absolutely appalling, because

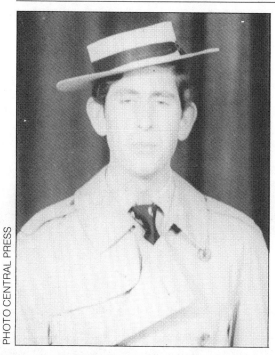

PHOTO CENTRAL PRESS

acting techniques – I mean timing and double entendres and everything are enormously helpful.

I enjoy making people laugh if I can and I always believe humour is a very useful way of getting people to listen to what you are saying.

In a sketch written by himself, Charles came onstage with an umbrella:
I lead a sheltered life.

Reading.

I have a congenital defect, which is being unable to remain awake for very long once I sit down with a book. But I do love reading very much and used to do a lot of it when I was at sea and had more time.

I tend to read a lot of history and a lot of biographies.

I'm fascinated by some of the books of Alexander Solzhenitsyn. I found 'The Gulag Archipelago' riveting, utterly horrifying and most moving.

Many people accused Solzhenitsyn of exaggeration, and maintained things were not nearly as bad as he made out. There will always be people like that.

Personally, I doubt that Solzhenitsyn is exaggerating when he talks about a decline in courage being possibly the most striking feature which an outside observer notices in the West in our days.

It does indeed seem as though one of the great abiding problems of Western society is the lack of individual courage of the sort that can withstand the fashionable attitudes of the pressures of collectivism.

According to Solzhenitsyn, we operate at the extreme limits of the legal framework of our societies, and he criticises the situation, saying, "Whenever the tissue of life is woven of legalistic relations there is an attitude of moral mediocrity paralysing man's noblest attitudes."

It's clear, I think, that we've neglected the moral factor in man. Karl Marx assumed that the goodness of man would assert itself automatically when the economic changes had been achieved.

when I finished there was a stunned silence from the parents until the producer in the wings started some applause.

In many places the facilities for amateur and professional acting are either non-existent or a disgrace to the community. Drama is just as important as gleaming new bingo halls, if not more so.

I can't help feeling it is an element of frustration and boredom which creates some of the uncivilised and uncouth reaction in present society and perhaps the theatre can absorb some of the frustration.

The Government is more than justified in spending money on the dramatic arts, and I hope they will continue to go on doing so.

To my regret, when I leave Cambridge the opportunities for acting, for crouching in uncollected dustbins and receiving custard pies in an ecclesiastical face, will be limited.

I love imitating and mimicking. I enjoyed acting enormously at school and university. In a strange way, so much of what one does requires acting ability one way or another and I enjoy it.

For instance, if you are making a speech it is extremely useful if you can use

But he didn't see that a better society couldn't be brought into life by people who hadn't undergone a moral change within themselves.

I think it's essential to consider the human aspects, and to examine industrial society from the standpoint of what it does to the human qualities of man, to his soul and his spirit.

Writing.

Charles made his début as a book reviewer by reviewing Harry Secombe's novel 'Twice Brightly' for Punch:

It is a compendium of Welsh wit and thespianism.

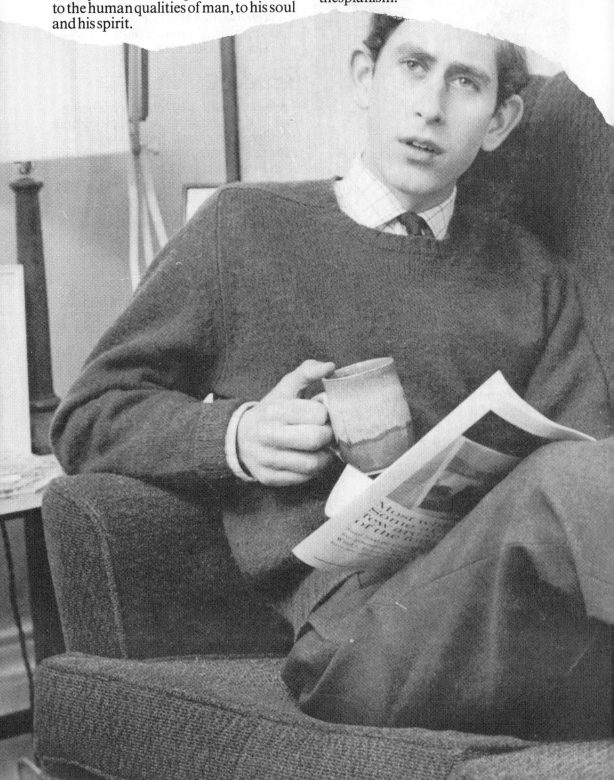

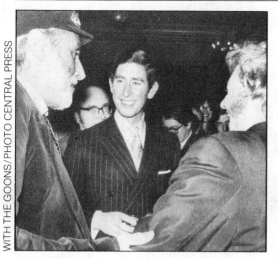

WITH THE GOONS./PHOTO CENTRAL PRESS

It reeks of the theatre, conjures up the excitement, the sheer knee-trembling terror of a first appearance on stage.

Charles loved The Goons and wrote an introduction to a volume of 'Goon Show' scripts:

It has always been one of my profound regrets that I was not born ten years earlier, since I would then have had the pure, unbounded joy of listening avidly to the Goons each week.

Instead, I only discovered that the Goon-type humour appealed to me just as the shows were drawing to a close. Then, I discovered 'The Ying Tong Song' in record form and, almost at once, I knew it by heart – the only song I do know by heart.

I plagued everybody with its dulcet tones and 'Solo For Raspberry Blower' to such an extent that when my small brothers heard a recording of the Goons for the first time they thought it was their elder brother!

It must be such hell writing a book. They are so *long,* aren't they?

I am hopelessly biased in favour of the works of Ned of Wales. I have always been an ardent supporter of this particular Welshman.

Reading the book, I was shaken with spasms of mirth at frequent intervals.

IN HIS STUDY AT CAMBRIDGE/PHOTO CENTRAL PRESS

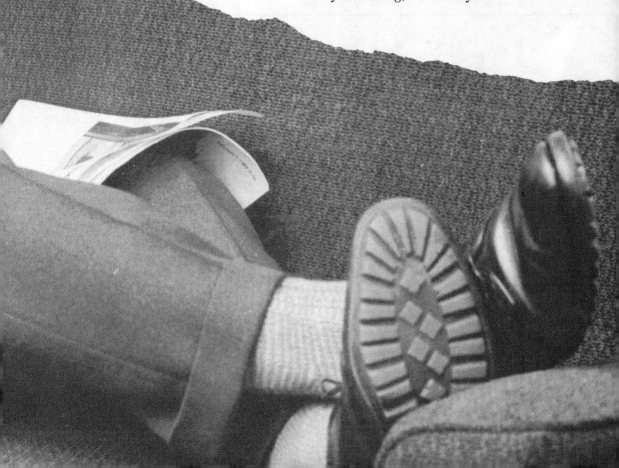

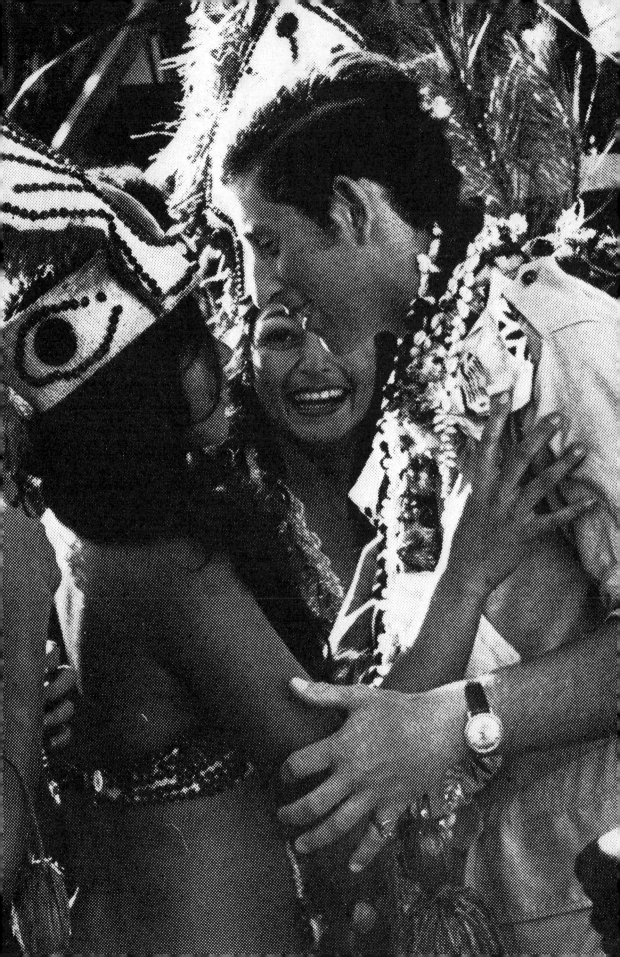

Travel.

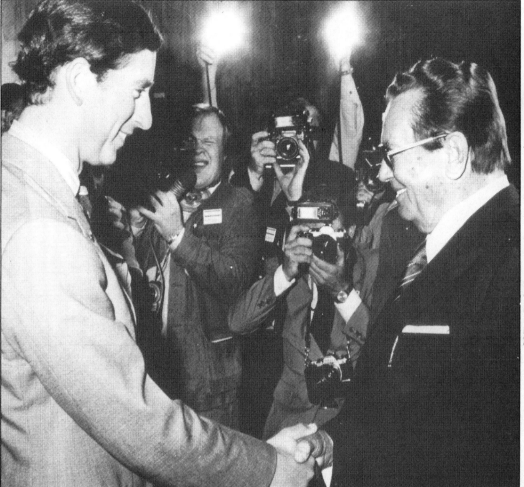

The whole idea of these visits is for me to meet as many people as I can, so they can see for themselves that I'm a pretty ordinary sort of person and not different from anyone else.

I hope that if I do go abroad, I can combine it with visiting various places and being a kind of ambassador.

My idea of a holiday is to do all the things I can't do when I'm not on holiday.

Many people think of a holiday as an occasion on which to lie down, go to sleep and do absolutely nothing. I like going off and being energetic, running around in circles and generally appearing absolutely mad.

I like going off somewhere really wild and seeing it before it has lodges built all over it.

Australia:

A funny thing happened to me on my way to Australia – I made a mistake and got off the plane.

The Australians:

They were very, very good and marvellous people. Very genuine, and said exactly what they thought. The only person who took the mickey out of me, or

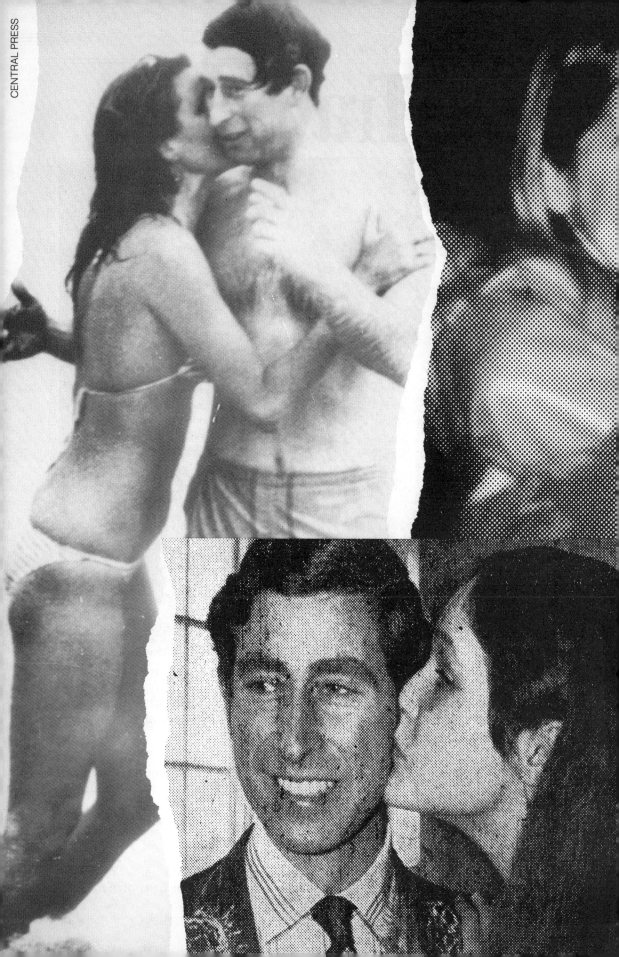

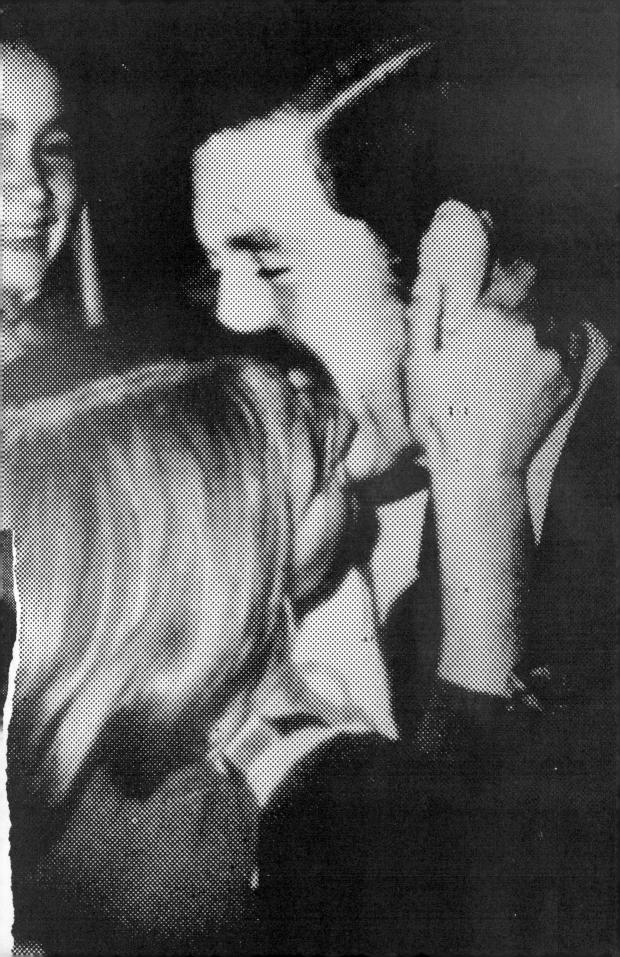

made me feel at all unhappy, I think, was an Englishman ... very strange, but that was the only time.

Except on another occasion when I went into the unit one evening and I had an umbrella with me – it had been raining quite heavily – and they all looked rather quizzically at this strange, English thing. As I walked out having turned the lights off, there were marvellous shouts of, "Oh, Pommy Bastard."

But that was about the only time the Australians ever took the mickey out of me, I think.

Arriving in Canberra in 1977:

I would like to meet as many people as possible during my stay, and this does not exclude eligible young ladies.

On renaming Brisbane's Chermside Hospital, Prince Charles Hospital:

I look forward to returning one day and naming it something else.

In the gold-mining city of Bendigo, huge crowds waited to see him:

It looks as though you have emptied out some of the pubs. However, I trust you won't waste good drinking time once I've gone into the town hall.

Charles first visited Papua during his first term at Timbertop in January 1966:

I can't help feeling that less and less interest is being taken by the younger Papuans in the customs and skills of their parents and grandparents. They feel that they have to live up to European standards and that these things belong to the past and have no relevance to the present or future.

This may be a completely false impression, but I was given one or two presents by young people and when I

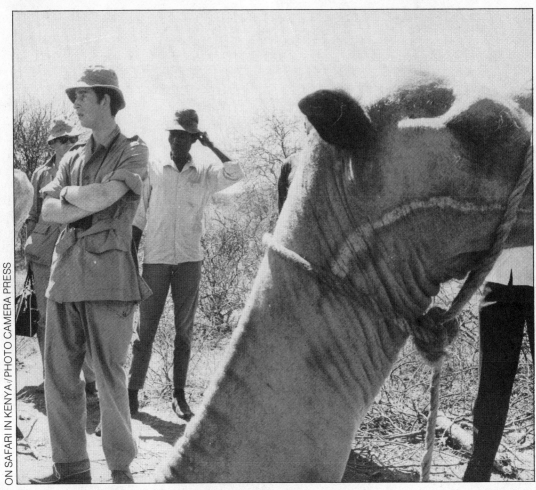

ON SAFARI IN KENYA/PHOTO CAMERA PRESS

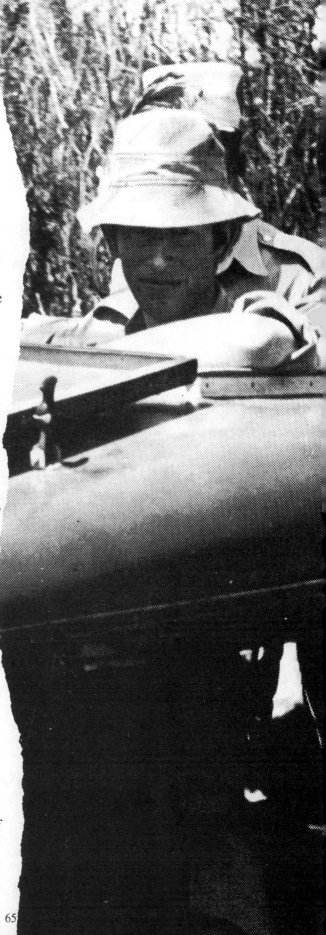

asked them if they had made them, they said their mothers or aunts had.

But I expect there will always be those who make souvenirs for tourists. If not, I hope a suitable amount of relics will be preserved for history.

I would like to mention how fresh and sincere I found the church at Dogura. Everyone was so eager to take part in the services, and the singing was almost deafening. One felt it might almost be the original church.

Where Christianity is new, it must be much easier to enter into the spirit of it wholeheartedly, and it is rather wonderful that you can still go somewhere where this strikes you.

Charles returned to Papua in 1975 for their independence ceremony. One of the islands was threatening to break away and Charles advised by quoting St. Paul's Epistle to the Romans:

"Everyone must obey the State authorities, for no authority exists without God's permission, and the existing authorities have been put there by God.

"Whoever opposes the existing authority opposes what God has ordered, and anyone who does so will bring judgement on himself."

Charles visited Bermuda in October 1970, as part of the island's celebration of 350 years of parliamentary government:

Bearing in mind that I am the first Charles to have anything to do with a Parliament for 350 years, I might have turned nasty and dissolved you.

Charles visited the Gilbert & Ellice Islands when they became independent. He was serving on the frigate Minerva at the time.

I am delighted to be here to escape from the clutches of my senior officers.

Charles and Anne visited Kenya on safari in February 1971:

That was something I really enjoyed. It was the best thing I've ever done, or one of the best – the sort of enlightened masochism which I go in for. The fun of it is one could really walk about the bush

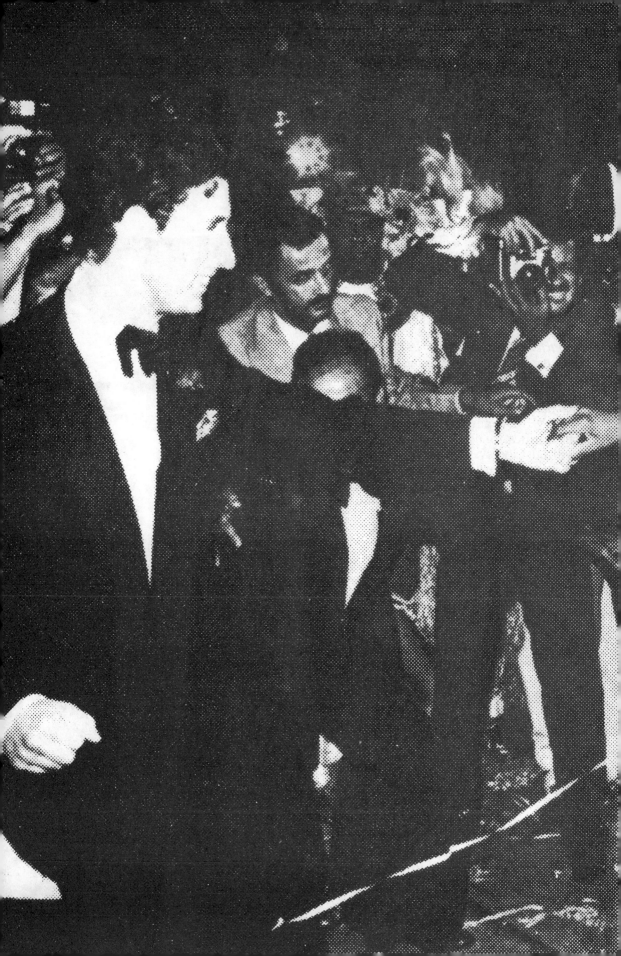

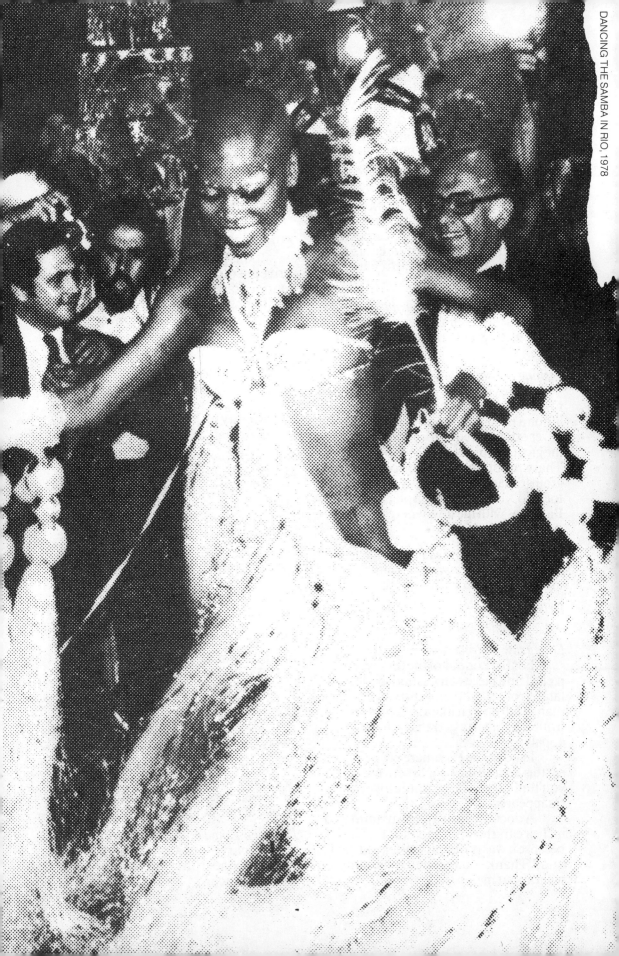

and come across animals suddenly and watch them.

The game scouts all thought I was absolutely mad, being in a dried-up piece of country instead of sitting in hotels and letting the animals come to me.

The first rhino seen is always a very exciting thing because they are prehistoric, primeval creatures and this one was just sort of standing there churning up the dust. Then it came closer and we were trying to see if we could get it to come closer still or perhaps charge us. But it didn't.

Visiting the Alhambra in Granada, 1972:
It's so marvellous, I can't understand why tourists don't take it away stone by stone.

Visiting Nassau in July 1973:
It provided me with the opportunity to discover the peace and fascination of life on a Bahamian beach – something I'd never experienced before and which gave me great happiness and contentment. That is, until I discovered those proverbial grains of sand wedged between the royal toes. So, you see, I carry a piece of the Bahamas with me now wherever I go.

Visiting Malta:
I am told many Maltese believe my future appearance was determined whilst my parents were on this island.

Driving a team of huskies in Canada:
That just sleighed me.

Eating raw seal meat with Eskimos:
For the honour of the family, I picked up a piece of meat and made the fatal error, of course, of chewing it rather than swallowing it like a sheep's eye. The trouble is that it tasted absolutely appalling.

I said, "The Press here are going to eat this, and all the people with me... you'll all eat it." They shrank away and disappeared.

A doctor who was with us muttered in their ears that they shouldn't eat it because it was probably a week old. So I said, "Thank you very much chummy, what about me, eh?!"

While in Canada, Charles dressed in Caribou fur:
I hope we don't meet a polar bear because he might think I'm in season.

Eskimos protested when Charles said:
I must be very careful as to whose nose I rub.

Charles later apologised:
I suppose it was a bad joke, a bad cliché. I hope I didn't give offence.

Zaire, 1979:
It was pouring with rain when I arrived at the airport. They had a guard of honour drawn up and they were absolutely soaked, poor things. I don't know why they didn't move them into a hangar. Next morning when I left, they were still there, soaked to the skin.

Ivory Coast, 1977:
Please be indulgent if I massacre the French language. I hope I may have the opportunity to find, perhaps, a brilliant Ivorian female teacher.

After spending several days in the Himalayan foothills of Nepal, 1980:
It was great fun. Each village turned out to greet us – everyone was so welcoming.

It was marvellous to wake up in the morning, open the tent window and see the mountains framed like a picture.

After hiking in the mountains:
Do I look disgusting enough? I'm not tired. I could still go on for three or four days.

India, November 1980:
As you know, in Britain we have welcomed many of your relatives.

During the same visit:
May the udders of your buffaloes be always full of milk.

Visiting the Taj Mahal, he was asked if he was touched by it:
Well, I did bang my head against the ceiling at one point.

Describing the Taj Mahal to the BBC:
A marvellous idea, to build something so wonderful... to someone one loved so much.

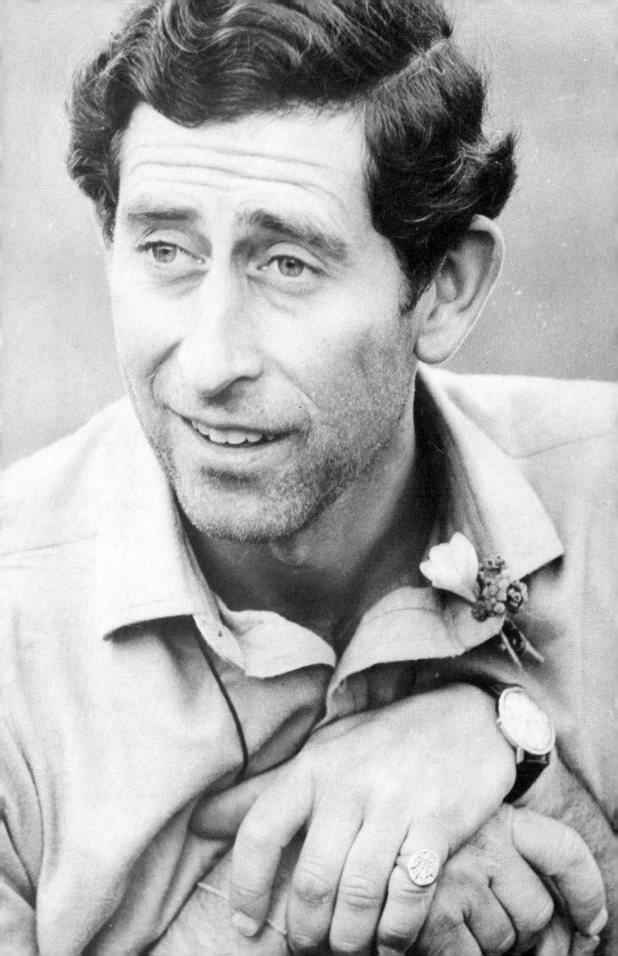

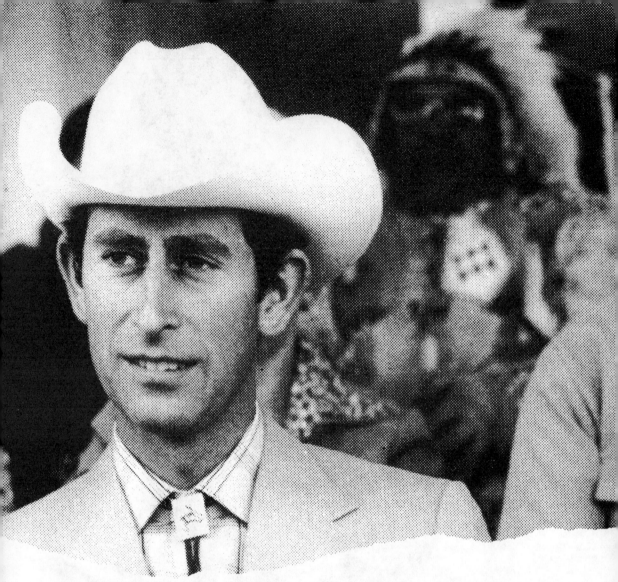

Speaking with an Indian actress in Bombay about her latest film:

Are there any bed scenes? No kissing either, I suppose.

About a girl he met in Texas in 1977:

I told her I'd like to make a sporting tour of America. She said to me, "Indoors or outdoors?" My reply is not on record.

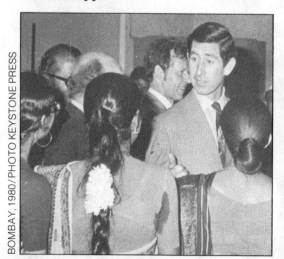

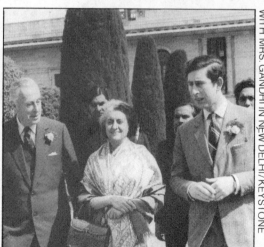

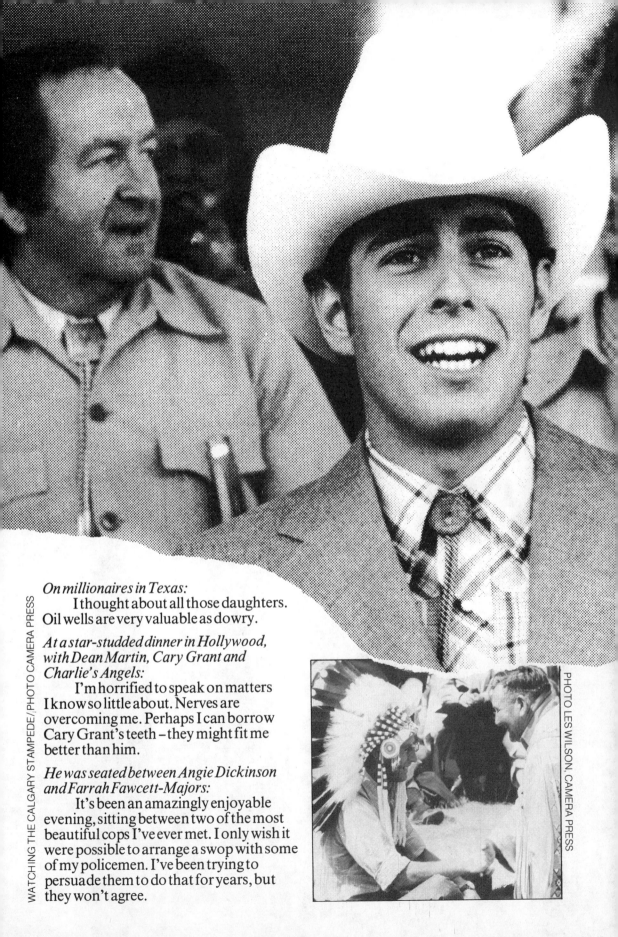

WATCHING THE CALGARY STAMPEDE./PHOTO CAMERA PRESS

On millionaires in Texas:

I thought about all those daughters.
Oil wells are very valuable as dowry.

*At a star-studded dinner in Hollywood,
with Dean Martin, Cary Grant and
Charlie's Angels:*

I'm horrified to speak on matters
I know so little about. Nerves are
overcoming me. Perhaps I can borrow
Cary Grant's teeth – they might fit me
better than him.

*He was seated between Angie Dickinson
and Farrah Fawcett-Majors:*

It's been an amazingly enjoyable
evening, sitting between two of the most
beautiful cops I've ever met. I only wish it
were possible to arrange a swop with some
of my policemen. I've been trying to
persuade them to do that for years, but
they won't agree.

PHOTO LES WILSON, CAMERA PRESS

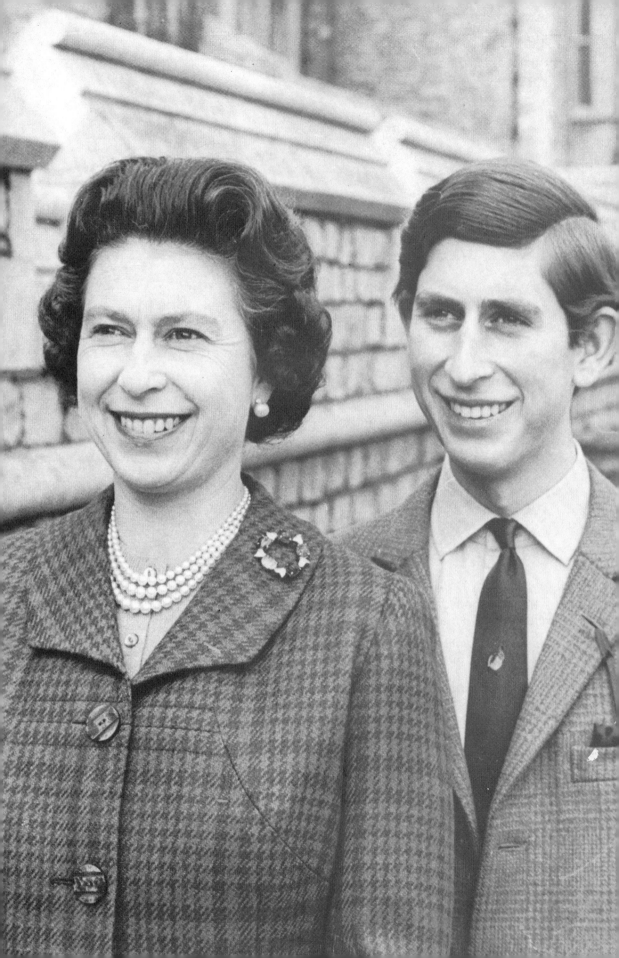

Family, Friends & Others.

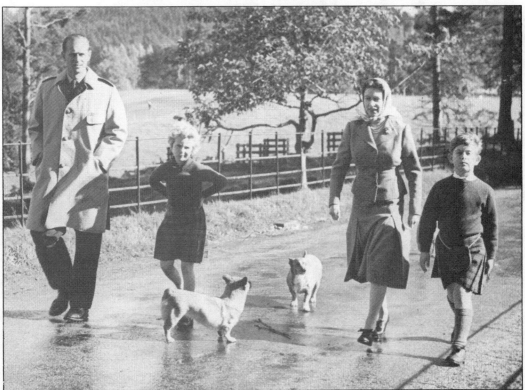

AT BALMORAL/PHOTO CENTRAL PRESS

The Royal Family:
It's like living in a glass-house.

I'm very lucky because I have very wise and incredibly sensible parents who have created a marvellous, secure, happy home.

I believe that the family unit is the most important aspect of our particular society. Above all else, it ensures that the majority of people are subject to an influence and an atmosphere of love, security – sanctions if you like – which are individual, rather than State-orientated.

I think the moment the family unit breaks down, it increases the chance of totalitarianism coming into operation.

I think, inevitably, some discipline is needed for children, and I think a lot of people expect somebody else to do the disciplining for them. I know I needed discipline.

If being old-fashioned means fostering a good family atmosphere, then I'm proud to be old-fashioned and will certainly remain so.

We are a family of human beings, not a set of symbols, and I think everybody would want us to be real.

I think of my family as very special people. I've never wanted not to have a home life – to get away from home. I love my home life. We happen to be a very close-knit family. I'm happier at home with my family than anywhere else.

I find I'm becoming a bit more independent. I think I may be slightly late in developing. I'm not sure.

His mother, the Queen:
    She is just a marvellous person and a wonderful mother.

His father, Prince Philip:
    He lets one get on with what you want to do. He gives one the opportunity to do these things. He says: "We think it might be an idea; what do you think?" In that sense, he's been an influence – but a moderating influence and an influence of great wisdom.

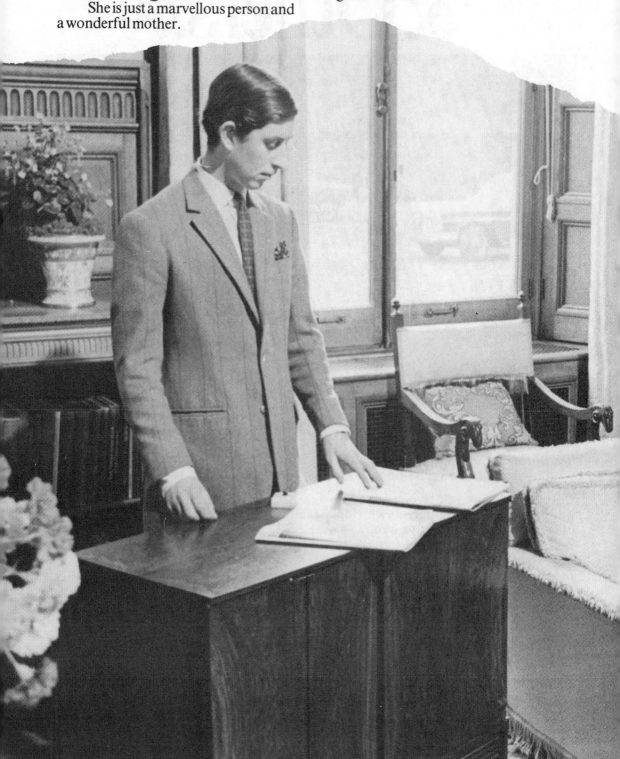

Charles and Philip no longer sail together:

I remember one disastrous day when we were racing and my father was, as usual, shouting. We wound the winch harder and the sail split in half with a sickening crack. Father was not pleased.

Not long after that, I was banned from the boat after an incident cruising in Scotland: There was no wind and I was amusing myself taking potshots at beer cans floating round the boat. The only gust of the day blew the jib in front of my rifle just as I fired. I wasn't invited back on board.

I'm often asked whether it's because of some generic trait that I stand with my hands behind my back, like my father. The answer is that we both have the same tailor – he makes the sleeves so tight that we can't get our hands in front.

The Queen Mother:

Ever since I can remember, my Grandmother has been the most wonderful example of fun, laughter, warmth, infinite security and, above all else, exquisite taste in so many things.

For me, she will always be one of those extraordinary, rare people whose touch can turn everything to gold – whether it be putting people at their ease, turning something dull into something

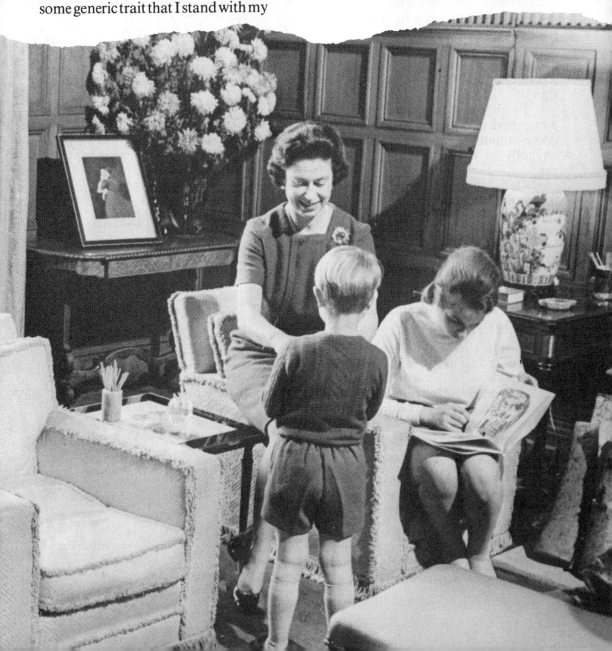

amusing, bringing happiness and comfort to people, or making any house she lives in a unique haven of cosiness and character.

Prince Andrew:
Ah, the one with the Robert Redford looks?

Lord Mountbatten:
He is a unique personality. In a way, he is the modern-day equivalent of Queen Victoria in relation to the family. He has the amazing ability to get on with everybody in the family.

He knows more about my immense family than anybody else. He has written relationship tables: he knows who everybody's related to as far back as... Charlemagne, on his side!

He also has an amazing ability for giving good advice, for sound reason, sensible and wise opinions about all things.

People love him because he is incredibly honest, straightforward, and doesn't mind what he says at all, to anybody and never has done from the year dot.

He is, I think, the centre of the family, the last person of his generation that knew everybody. He was brought up to think very strongly that the family was an important concept, which I feel very deeply too.

Certainly, Lord Mountbatten has had an influence on my life and I admire him, I think, almost more than anybody else. He's a very great person.

After Mountbatten was murdered:
I adored him – and miss him so dreadfully now.

It is a cruel and bitter irony that he should have survived two world wars and then be blown to bits by sub-human extremists.

He had that quality of real moral courage, of being able to tackle unpleasant tasks. That, in these days, is a rare quality indeed. He had it in abundance.

Prince Louis of Battenberg:
Pride swells when I recall the part played by my great-grandfather in the formation of the Royal Naval Air

WITH LORD MOUNTBATTEN

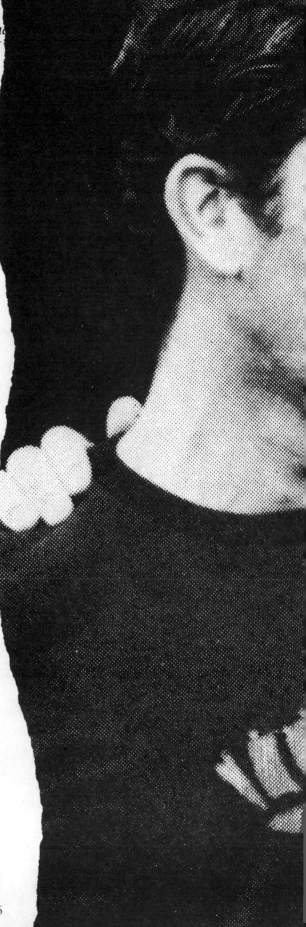

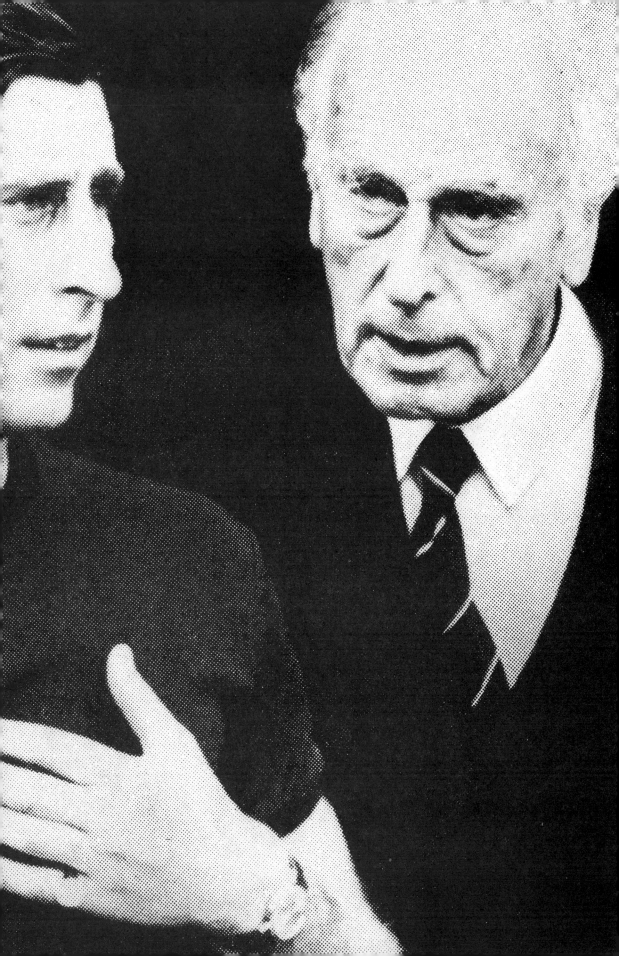

Squadron in 1914. Without his interest and enthusiasm, and his determined support of the aeroplane versus the airship, the Naval Air Service might quite literally have had great difficulty in getting off the ground.

Charles I:
I realised that Charles I was not entirely splendid and innocent, as I had always thought.

His ancestor, King George III:
I think I first got interested because people have gone on for years and years in the history books describing him as the

"mad Monarch." If you ask any school child, I'll bet you what he says about George III is that he was mad.

I felt that he was a much-maligned monarch – particularly by American historians who obviously found it convenient to blame him to a certain extent, to make it easier to justify the American Revolution. They could argue they were revolting against a mad monarch who had no credibility in America.

His so-called madness, in the light of modern medical knowledge and research, may in fact have resulted from a physical

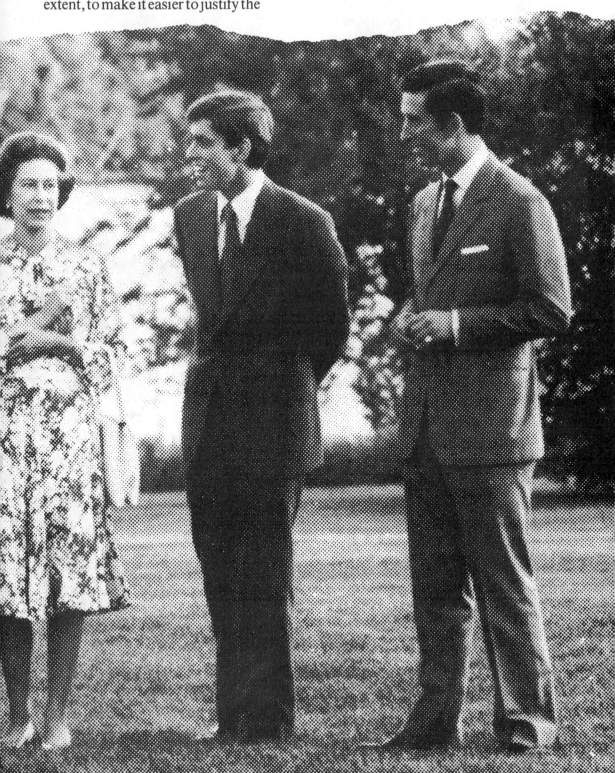

disease, a condition of the blood known as porphyria. This actually makes you appear demented occasionally; it goes in cycles.

He was a great patron of the arts, and a great patron of scientific development in the 18th century.

I admire him enormously for what he did and for his incredible capacity for hard work and conscientious devotion to duty.

A lot of people would regard this as boring because he didn't do what Charles II reportedly did and have affairs with all sorts of delectable ladies. That's always much more glamorous than a chap who works hard and is a conscientious monarch – and is also more discreet!

His friends:

I tend to have a few, but very good friends. I always rather fought shy, at school and elsewhere, of group or gang behaviour. I've always been happier with one or two people. I do have some marvellous friends – I'm very lucky. I've made them since I left school. I've just got one or two friends left that I knew at school.

I trust my friends implicitly, and they know that. The more discreet, the better. Those people who do get drawn into conversations and do natter about me find they get into the papers. But I hear they don't get paid very much. Five pounds, or two pounds. Or is it ten with inflation?

I do have friends outside a narrow circle; it's a different type of friendship. A person's closest friends, whatever his position, are determined by his interests and way of life. For instance, I enjoy shooting: therefore, I see a lot of people who shoot. A number of them are "members of the aristocracy." Not all. But it isn't that they are landed gentry which is the *cause* of my seeing them. It's shooting.

On the other hand, when I was at Cambridge, I got to know some very different kinds of people. One man in particular comes to mind, and he's an academic. We write to each other, but we don't meet as often as we did because he's in the North of England and I'm down

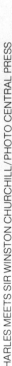

here. The fact that I don't "mix" with him as much as I did isn't because he's a different kind of person, or because he comes from a different "class" – it's a matter of circumstance.

Winston Churchill:
His recorded words still cause a tingle to run up and down my spine and bring a tear to my eye. He was able to use words the way Mozart used musical notes.

There is a loch in the grounds called Loch Muick which we used to net for trout. I've never forgotten seeing him seated on a rock in the loch with an enormous tree trunk across his knees saying, "I am waiting for the Loch Muick monster."

Frank Sinatra:
Sinatra could be terribly nice one minute, and, well, not so nice, the next. I was not impressed with the creeps and mafia types he kept around him.

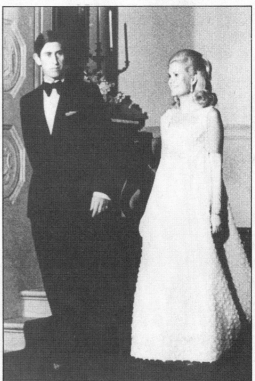

WITH TRICIA NIXON/PHOTO JAMES PICKERELL, CAMERA PRESS

Tricia Nixon:
Artificial and plastic.

Julie Nixon:
A bright, warm personality.

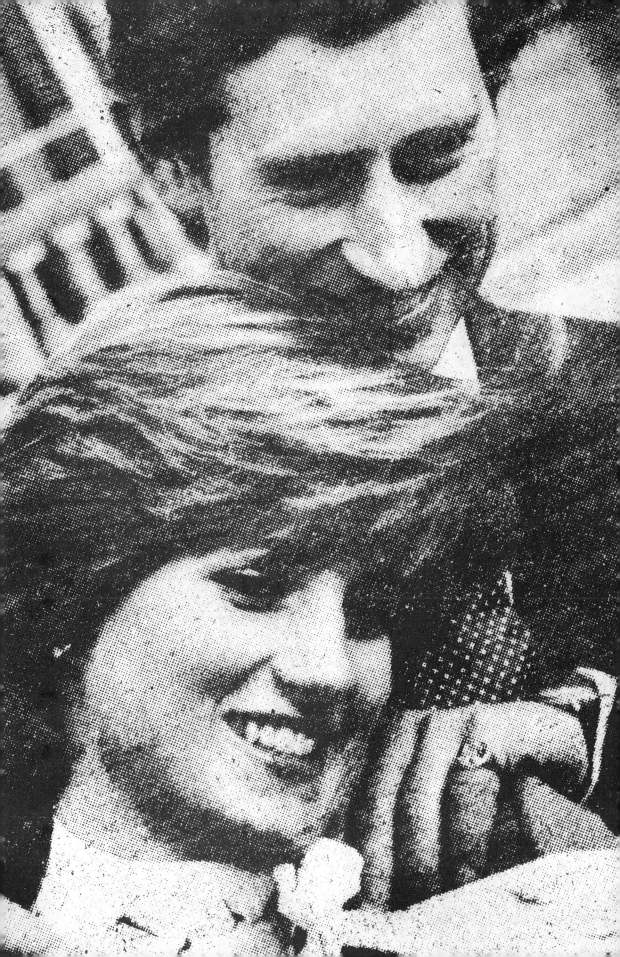

Love & Marriage.

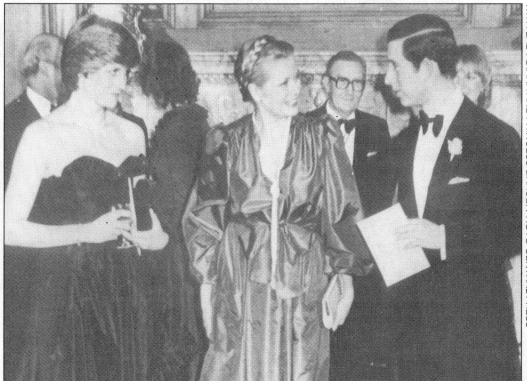

A lot of people, I feel, have a false idea about love. I think it's more than just a romantic idea of falling madly in love with someone and having a love affair for the rest of your life. It's much more than that: it's a very strong friendship.

As often as not, you have shared interests and ideas in common, plus a great deal of affection. You are very lucky when you find someone who attracts you in the physical, as well as the mental sense.

Obviously, there must be someone, somewhere for me.

When you get to my extraordinary stage of decrepitude, you begin to think about things like that, as I'm sure you know. You look at a girl and think, "I wonder if one could ever marry her," or something like that.

And obviously, there are certain people I've thought of on those lines.

In many cases, one falls madly in "love" with somebody with whom you are infatuated rather than in love.

I hope I will be as lucky as my own parents who have been so happy.

His Ladies.

It's very hard on them, I have layers to protect me, but they are not used to it. It tends, sometimes, to put the really nice

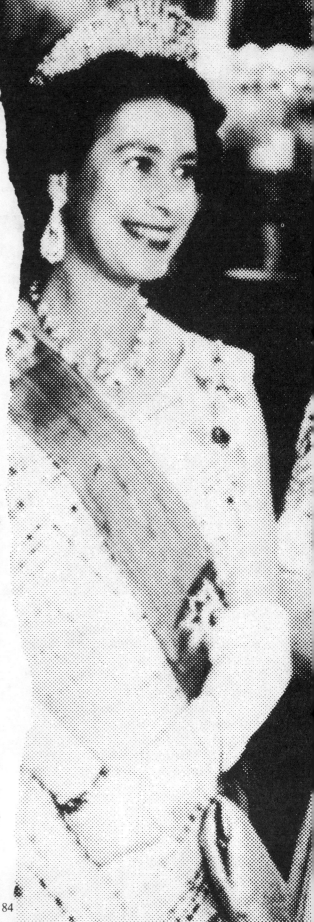

ones off. Poor Jane Wellesley; I am
shielded, but how can she be protected?

Lady Jane Wellesley:
There was also that marvellous
theory that the reason for Princess Anne's
marriage was to allow me to conduct my
operations under cover. Of course,
nothing transpired.

But as you know, only too well, the
great problem as a result of my sister
announcing her engagement, having said
only a few months previously that there
was no truth in the rumours is that the
Press, I know, will never, ever again,
believe it if you say there is no truth and
we're just good friends!

Princess Caroline of Monaco:
I have only met the girl once and they
are trying to marry us off.

Princess Marie-Astrid:
If I marry a Catholic, I'm dead. I've
had it.

Marriage.

Referring to Edward VIII:
I will not become a martyr to the
cause.

Whenever I give a dinner party these days,
more and more of the people seem to be
married.

Marriage is a much more important
business than falling in love. I think one
must concentrate on marriage being
essentially a question of mutual love and
respect for each other.

Creating a secure family unit in
which to bring up children, to give them a
happy, secure upbringing – that's what
marriage is all about, creating a home.

Essentially, you must be good
friends, and love, I'm sure, will grow out
of that friendship.

I have a particular responsibility to
ensure that I make the right decision. The
last thing I could possibly entertain is
getting divorced.

I've fallen in love with all sorts of girls
and I fully intend to go on doing so. But,
I've made sure I haven't married the first
person I've fallen in love with.

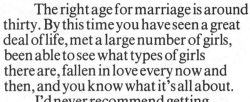

The right age for marriage is around thirty. By this time you have seen a great deal of life, met a large number of girls, been able to see what types of girls there are, fallen in love every now and then, and you know what it's all about.

I'd never recommend getting married too young. You miss so much, you get tied down.

I certainly won't get married until I've left the Navy. I couldn't cope with both. It would be too difficult a problem, and I think it's very unfair on a woman to be continually left behind. I'd rather wait until I could supply as much company as possible, particularly in the first years of marriage.

I like to think I've watched other people. Having tried to learn from other people's experiences, other people's mistakes – yes, in one's own family and in other people's – I hope I shall be able to make a reasonable decision and choice.

The more industrialised and artificial our lives become, the more standards tend to fall. I think one of the reasons the divorce rate goes up is because people no longer feel that marriage is important.

You have to remember that when you marry in my position, you're going to marry someone who, perhaps, is one day going to be queen. You've got to choose somebody very carefully, I think, who could fulfil this particular role, and it has got to be somebody pretty unusual.

The one advantage about marrying a princess, for instance, or somebody from a royal family, is that they do know what happens.

The only trouble is that I often feel I'd like to marry somebody English, or, perhaps, Welsh. Well, British anyway.

To me, marriage – which may be for fifty years – seems to be one of the biggest and most responsible steps to be taken in one's life. Which makes it all sound hideously complicated.

My marriage has to be for ever. It's sad, in a way, that some people should feel that there is every opportunity to just break it off when you feel like it. I mean,

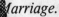

the whole point about the marriage contract was that it was for life.

And marriage isn't only for the two people who form the marriage; it's also for the children of that marriage.

Presumably, in the first place, the institution of marriage was started in order to allow children to have a reasonable degree of security in their upbringing so that they became reasonable and responsible human beings. But if they were the children of people who simply dashed from one place to another with different people all the time, they'd turn into the most extraordinary individuals – as happens only too often.

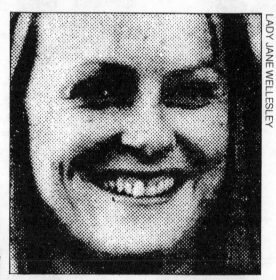

LADY JANE WELLESLEY

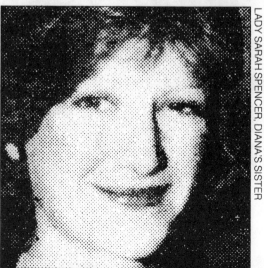

LADY SARAH SPENCER, DIANA'S SISTER

If you feel you can change it, change your mind and try anybody else at the drop of a hat, then that's sad. Marriage is something you ought to work at. I may easily be proved wrong, but I certainly intend to work at it when I get married.

Whatever your place in life, when you marry you're forming a partnership which you hope will last, say, fifty years. I certainly hope so, because I've been brought up in a close-knit, happy family, and family life means more to me than anything else. So I'd want to marry somebody who had interests which I understood and could share.

Then look at it from the woman's point of view. A woman not only marries a man, she also marries into a way of life, into a job, into a life in which she's got a contribution to make. She's got to have some knowledge of it, some sense of it, or she wouldn't have a clue about whether she's going to like it. If she didn't have a clue, it would be too risky for her, wouldn't it?

If I'm deciding on whom I want to live with for the next fifty years – well that's the last decision in which I'd want my head to be ruled entirely by my heart. It's nothing to do with class; it's to do with compatibility.

There are as many cases of marriages turning out unsatisfactorily because a man married above himself as there are

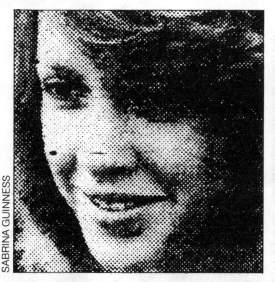

SABRINA GUINNESS

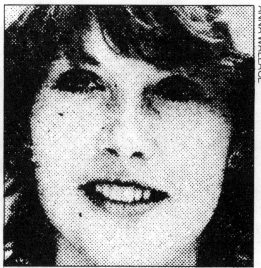

ANNA WALLACE

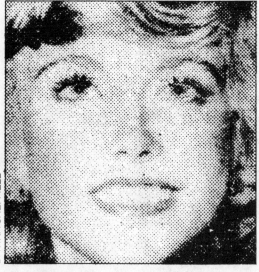

DAVINA SHEFFIELD

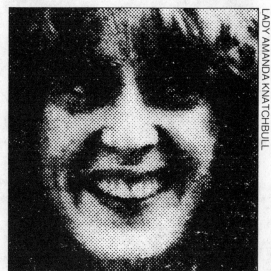

LADY AMANDA KNATCHBULL

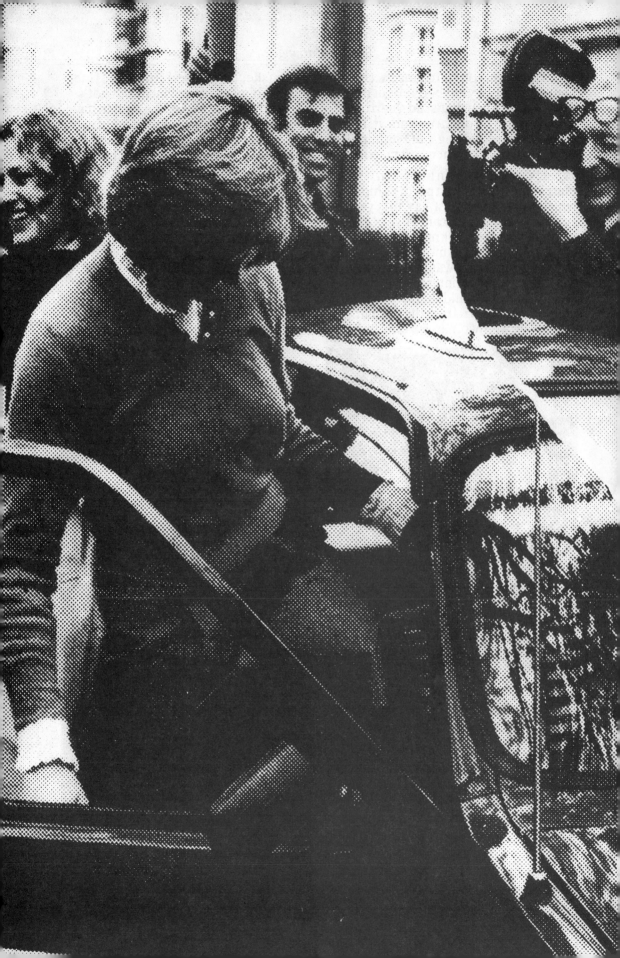

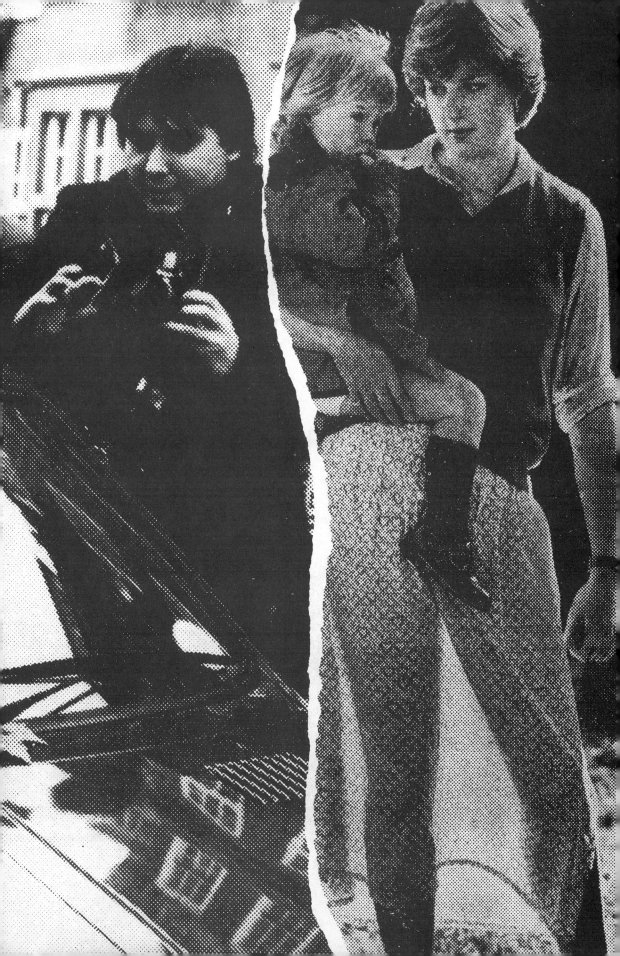

CHEVENING HOUSE IN KENT/PHOTO A.F. KERSTING

when he married below. Marriage isn't an "up" or "down" issue anyway: it's a side-by-side one.

Lady Diana.

Diana was an old friend of the family. Charles remembered:
What a very amusing and jolly – and attractive – sixteen-year-old she was.

Diana is a real outdoor-loving sort of person.

Diana is a great skier.

They were together at Balmoral during July 1980:
I began to realise what was going on in *my* mind and hers in particular.

Charles confided to an aide during his walking tour in the Himalayas:
I'm terrified of getting it wrong.

Charles proposed over dinner for two in his third-floor quarters at Buckingham Palace before Diana went to Australia:
I wanted to give Diana a chance to think about it – to think if it all was going to be too awful.

She'd planned to go to Australia quite a long time before anyway, with her mother, and I thought, "Well, I'll ask her then so that she'll have a chance of thinking it over while she's away and saying, 'I can't bear the whole idea' – or not, as the case may be."

After his proposal was accepted:
I feel positively delighted and frankly amazed that Di is prepared to take me on.

Their honeymoon:
We've discussed vague ideas and now people might come up with suggestions of where we might go.

The difference between their ages:
I haven't somehow thought about it. I mean, it's only twelve years and lots of people have got married with that sort of age difference. I just feel you are as old as you think you are.

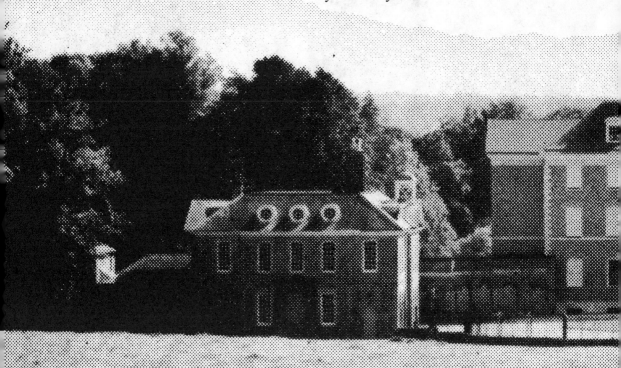

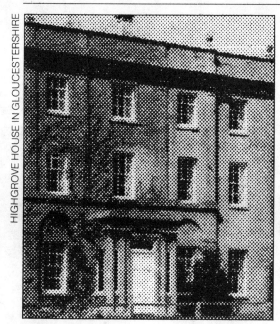

HIGHGROVE HOUSE IN GLOUCESTERSHIRE

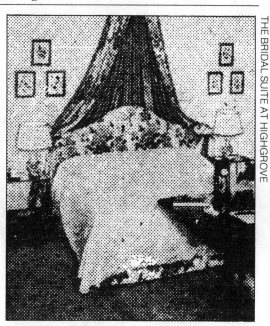

THE BRIDAL SUITE AT HIGHGROVE

Diana will certainly keep me young. I think I shall be exhausted.

Where to live:
I only have two rooms and a bedroom at the Palace, so it will obviously be difficult to stay here for very long.

Highgrove in Gloucestershire:
It will be marvellous to have someone to take it on and organise everything, because it's completely empty at the moment. I haven't moved in. I just camp there whenever I can.

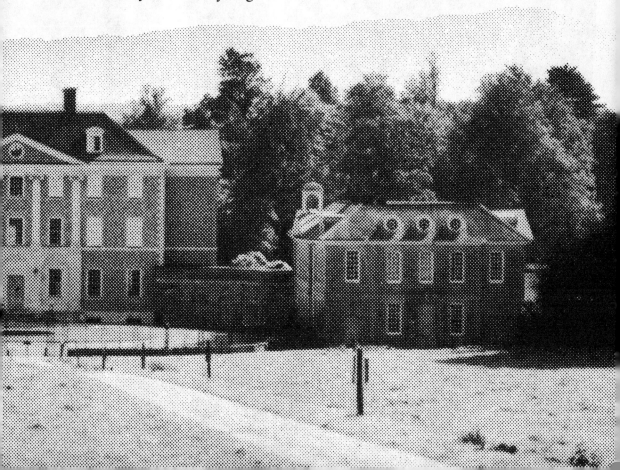

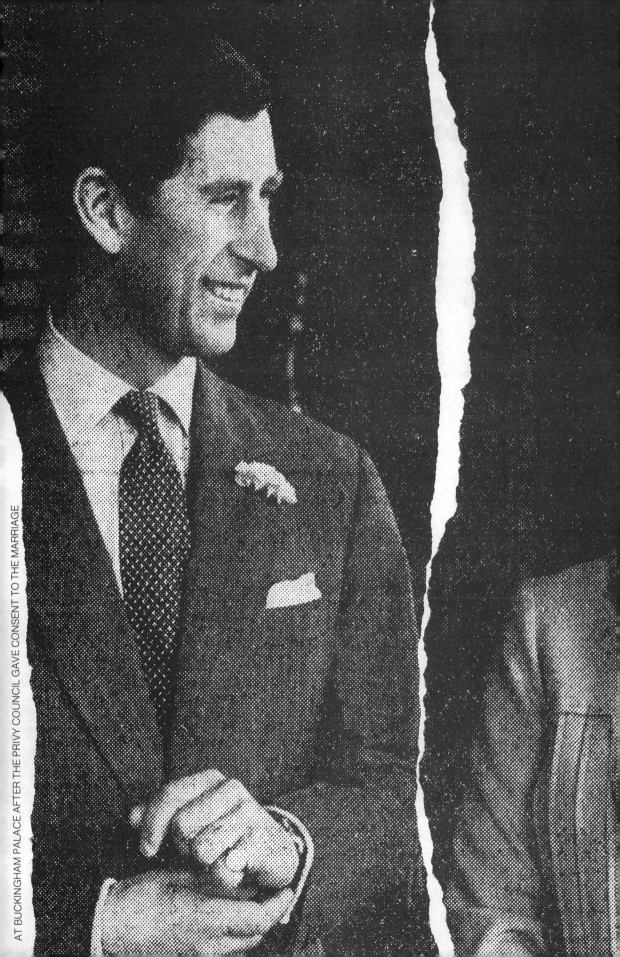

AT BUCKINGHAM PALACE AFTER THE PRIVY COUNCIL GAVE CONSENT TO THE MARRIAGE

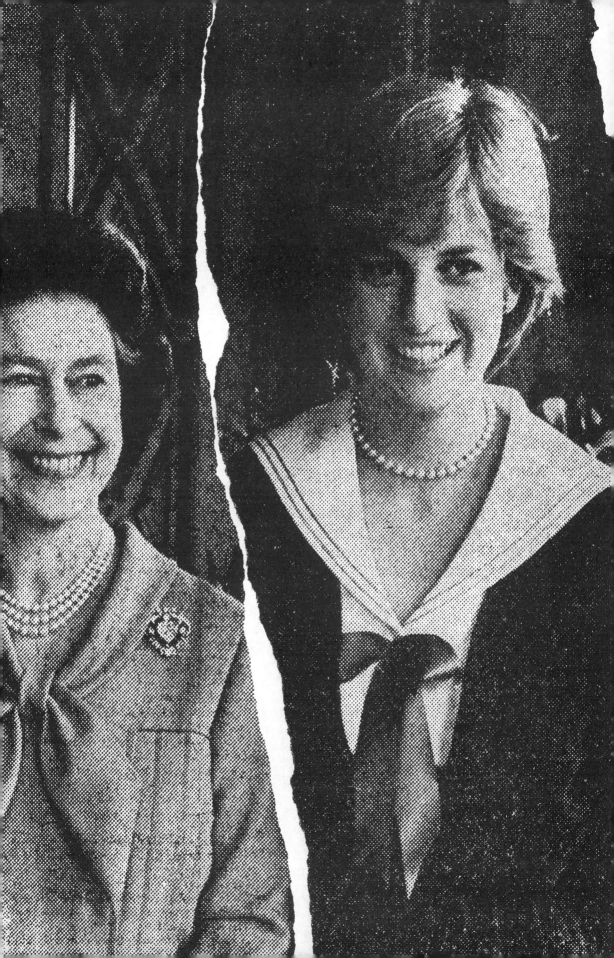

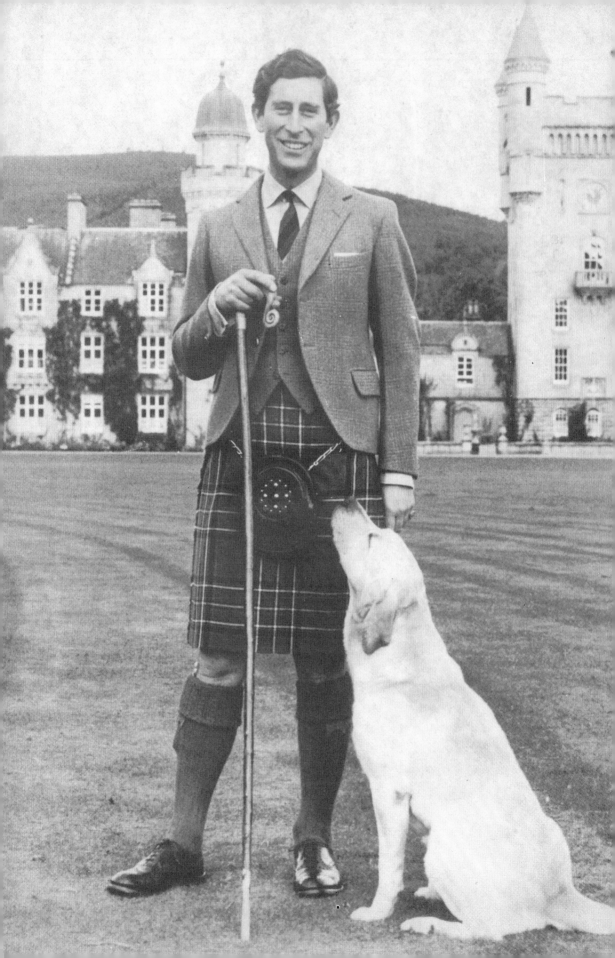

Charles On Himself.

I tend to be a jack-of-all-trades.

Were it not for my ability to see the funny side of my life, I'd have been committed to an institution long ago.

David Frost asked him how he'd describe himself:
Sometimes, a bit of a twit.

The most important quality a person like myself needs is a sense of humour and the ability to laugh at oneself.

When we've been talking at sea, some of the sailors say, "Wouldn't you like to have a life of your own? Wouldn't you like to be able to go down to the pub?" Well, I *have* got a life of my own, and I like it. Life doesn't consist of going down to the pub. The pleasure in life consists of going down to the pub if that's what you like to do.
And I do quite as much of what I like to do as is good for me, and I do a lot of other things which are work, just as everybody else has to work. Sometimes the sailors said, "Wouldn't you like to be free?" Free from what? Being free isn't doing what other people like to do, it's doing what *you* like to do.
I'm not a rebel by temperament. I don't get a kick out of not doing what is expected of me, or of doing what is not expected of me. I don't feel an urge to react against older people. I've been brought up with older people and I've enjoyed it. And now that I'm twenty-five, other people's ages don't matter anyway.

Occasionally you have to stick your neck out.

I was asked whether I concentrated on developing my "image" – as if I was some kind of washing powder, presumably with a special blue whitener. I have absolutely no idea what my image is and therefore I intend to go on being myself to the best of my ability.
I dare say that I could improve my image in some circles by growing my hair to a more fashionable length, being seen at the Playboy Club at frequent intervals, and squeezing myself into tight clothes.

I dare say many of my views and beliefs would be considered old-fashioned and out of date. But that doesn't worry me... Fashion, by its very definition, is transitory; human nature being what it is, what was old-fashioned at length becomes in fashion. Thus the whole process continues.

I don't believe in fashion, full stop. I admit I am pretty square. I couldn't care less.

Yes, I think one can be normal if one starts being an international personality right from the word go.

I'm not a normal person in the sense that I was born to be king. I've received a special education and training. I could never be a normal person because I've been prepared to reign over my subjects.

While making a speech, he touched on the problems of public speaking:
I can tell you that writing speeches is a major sweat. Actually sitting down and thinking is a sweat. Worrying whether you're going to say the right thing is another problem, of course, because everybody will jump on you.
You have no idea, ladies and gentlemen, what excruciating suffering you have caused, what intense intellectual effort has been expended upon this oration involving innumerable man hours

at a negative rate of overtime. Life, I can assure you, is tough at the top!

My profession is somewhat indefinable and so I find myself holding forth on subjects about which I know very little for far too long.

My views change and my outlook evolves as I grow older, and I deeply resent being attributed with views I expressed as a younger, and less wise man.

The problem is to get through a certain amount of anxiety or nervousness or prejudice, or whatever to start with. It usually takes about twenty minutes ...

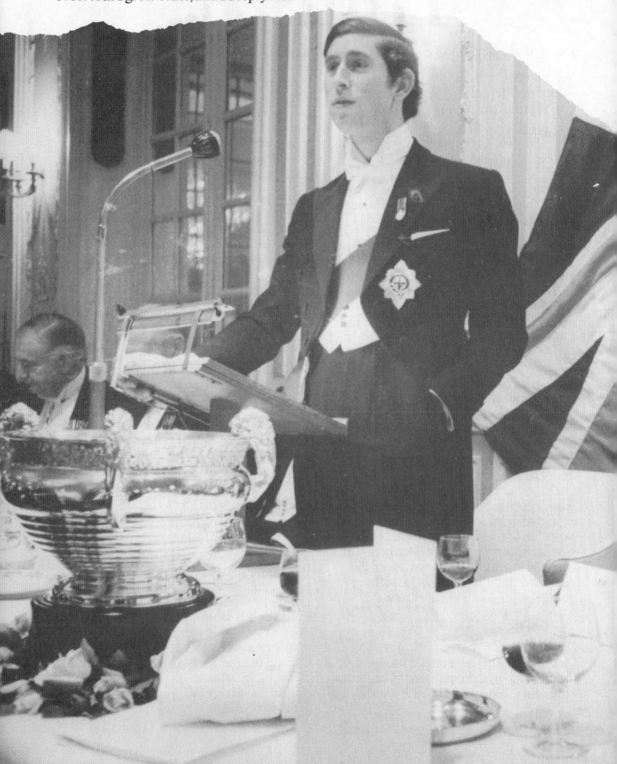

they're maybe beginning to realise that you're vaguely human and then you've got to go.

I'm still fairly shy. One just has to conquer this. It's one of those things that comes as you grow older.

I don't make friends all that easily. Perhaps the position that one is in builds up a little bit of a barrier, but I find now that I'm making more friends.

The time to get anxious, in a way, is when nobody's interested at all.

Many people are too shy and overcome in the presence of royalty. Only the dignitaries seem to talk to me on well-tried subjects, usually of little interest.

Unfortunately the nicest people are those who won't come up and make themselves known. They're terrified of being seen to be friendly in case they'll be accused of sucking-up or because they imagine, quite wrongly, that I won't want to talk to them.

I used to think, "Good God, what's wrong? Do I smell? Have I forgotten to change my socks?" I realise now that I have to make a bit of the running and show that I'm a reasonable human being. An awful lot of people say eventually, "Good Lord, you're not nearly as pompous as I thought you were going to be."

PHOTO KEYSTONE

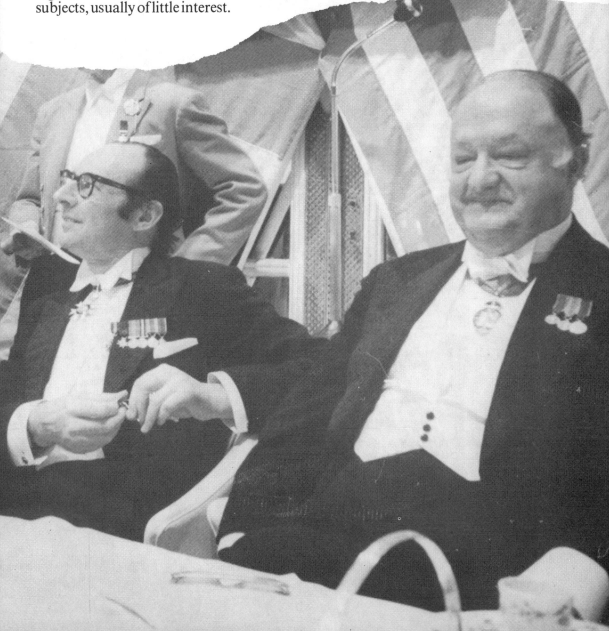

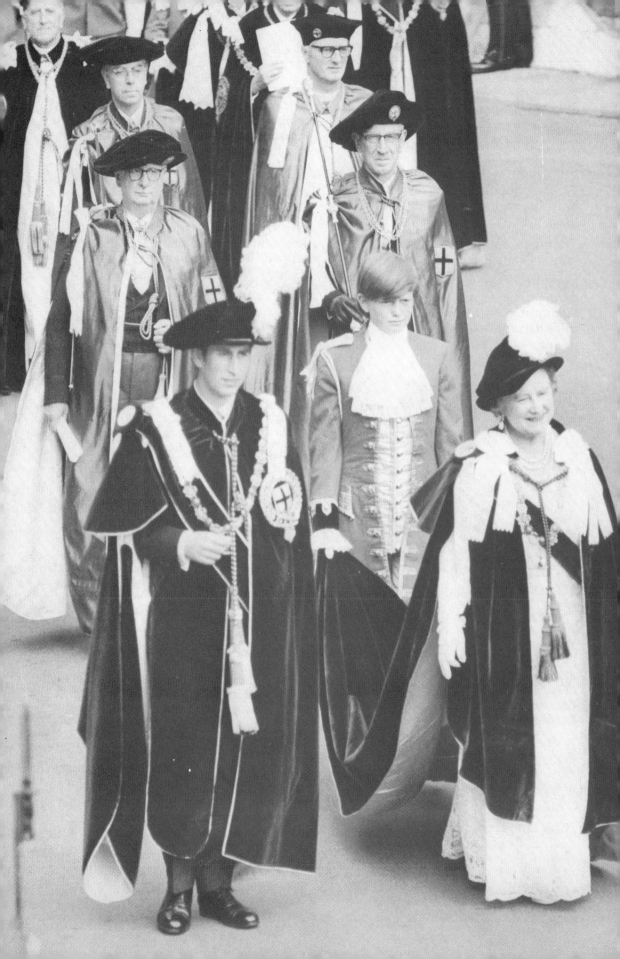

The Monarchy.

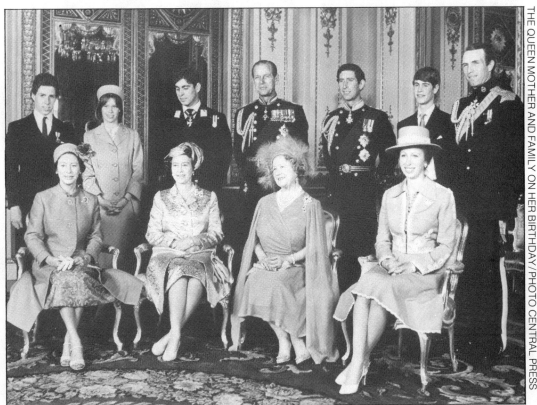

THE QUEEN MOTHER AND FAMILY ON HER BIRTHDAY/PHOTO CENTRAL PRESS

One of the oldest professions in the world.

I maintain that the greatest function of any monarchy is the human concern which its representatives have for the people, especially in what is becoming an increasingly inhuman era – an age of computers, machines, multi-national organisations. This, to my mind, is where the future can be promising.

In these times, the monarchy is called into question – it's not to be taken for granted as it used to be. In that sense, one now has to be far more professional.

I don't think monarchs should retire and be pensioned off, say, at sixty, as some professions and businesses stipulate. The nature of being a monarch is different.
    Take Queen Victoria. In her eighties she was more loved, more known, more revered in her country than she'd ever been before.
    In other walks of life too, age may bring accumulations of respect – and possibly wisdom – which are valuable to society. Looking at the monarchy as objectively as I can, I'd say retirement at a certain age is not a sensible idea. Some kind of unfitness is a different matter, but you must leave it to the monarch concerned.
    If you look outside this country, King Gustav of Sweden reigned until he was ninety. I think most people agree that Sweden would have lost something had he retired at sixty.

There isn't any power. But there can be influence. The influence is in direct proportion to the respect people have for you.

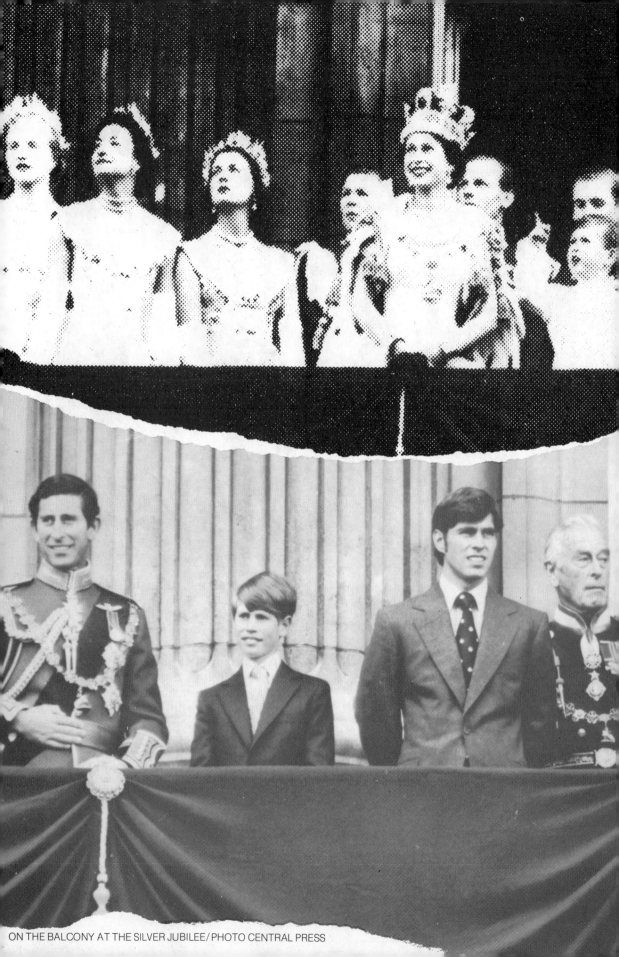

ON THE BALCONY AT THE SILVER JUBILEE/ PHOTO CENTRAL PRESS

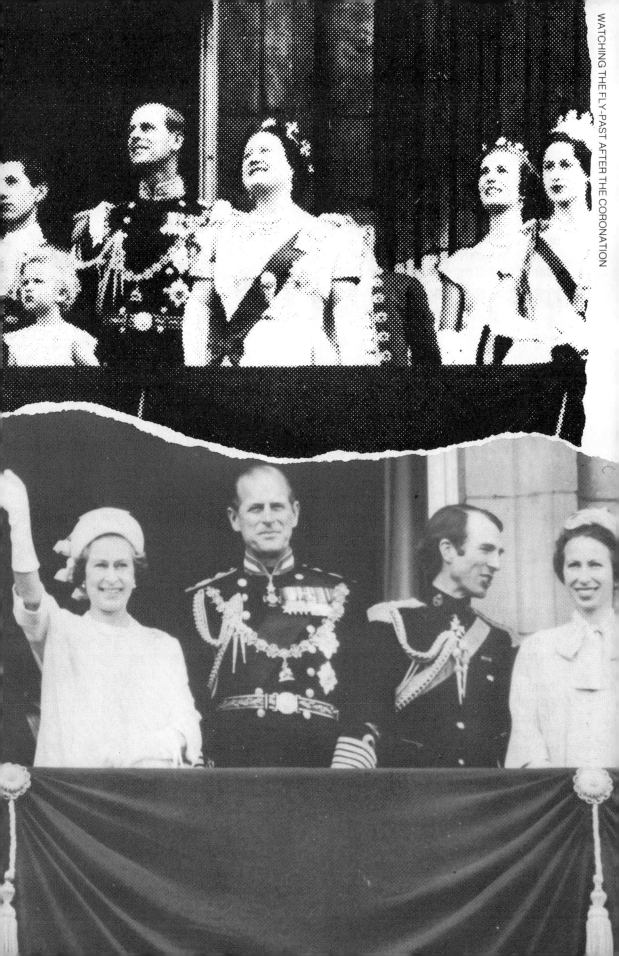

I'd change nothing. Besides ceremony being a major and important aspect of monarchy – something that has grown and developed over a thousand years in Britain – I happen to enjoy it enormously.

It's only right, I think, that in company with convicts, lunatics and peers of the realm, I'm ineligible to vote.

This is, of course, exactly as it should be: not necessarily in relation to convicts, but in relation to the monarchy.

The monarchy has done its best to adapt to changing circumstances, but

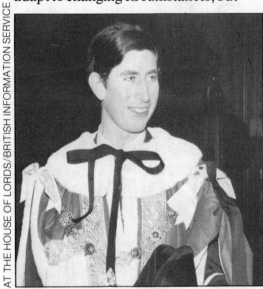

inevitably, it's more difficult to adapt when the accepted patterns of life and society are changing so unusually fast.

Monarchy is, I do believe, the system mankind has so far evolved which comes nearest to ensuring stable government.

I also believe that the institution of the monarchy – to which, rightly or wrongly, I belong and which I represent to the best of my ability – is one of the strongest factors in the continuance of stable government.

The Silver Jubilee.

It was great fun and, when done well and tastefully, there's nothing more marvellous than this sort of thing. Judging by the number of people in the streets, and their enthusiasm, they enjoyed it too.

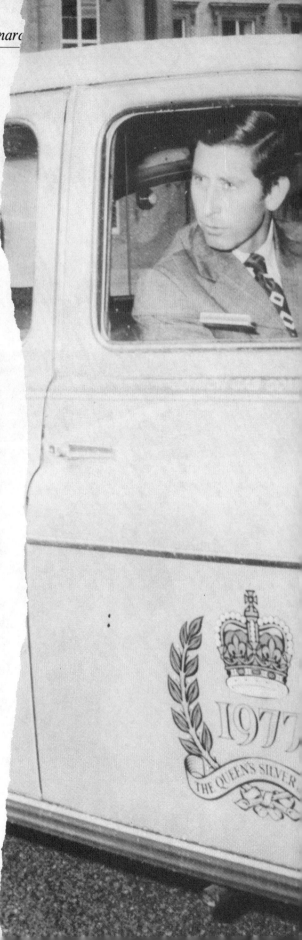

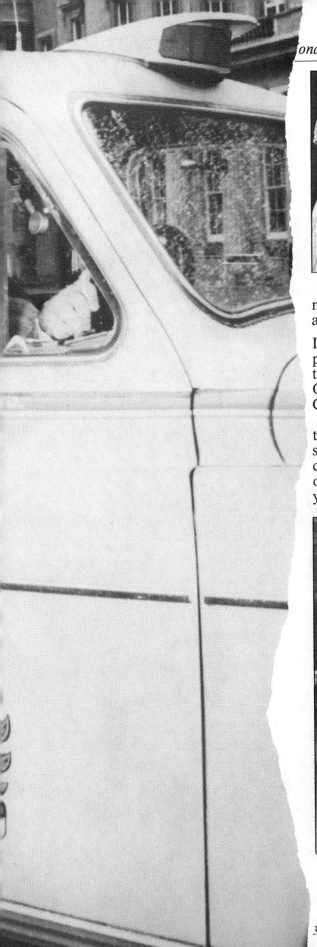

onarchy.

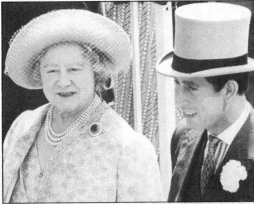

PHOTO CENTRAL PRESS

Apart from anything else it was the most wonderful expression of happiness and affection for the Queen.

I felt it'd be marvellous if there was some permanent way in which we could mark the twenty-five years of service which the Queen has given to the country and the Commonwealth.

I asked my mother what she'd like us to do. After careful consideration, she said she'd be particularly pleased if money could be raised to assist and encourage the outstanding work already being done by young people in various fields.

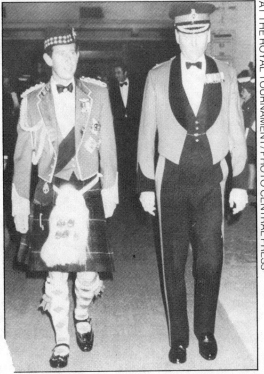

AT THE ROYAL TOURNAMENT/PHOTO CENTRAL PRESS

3

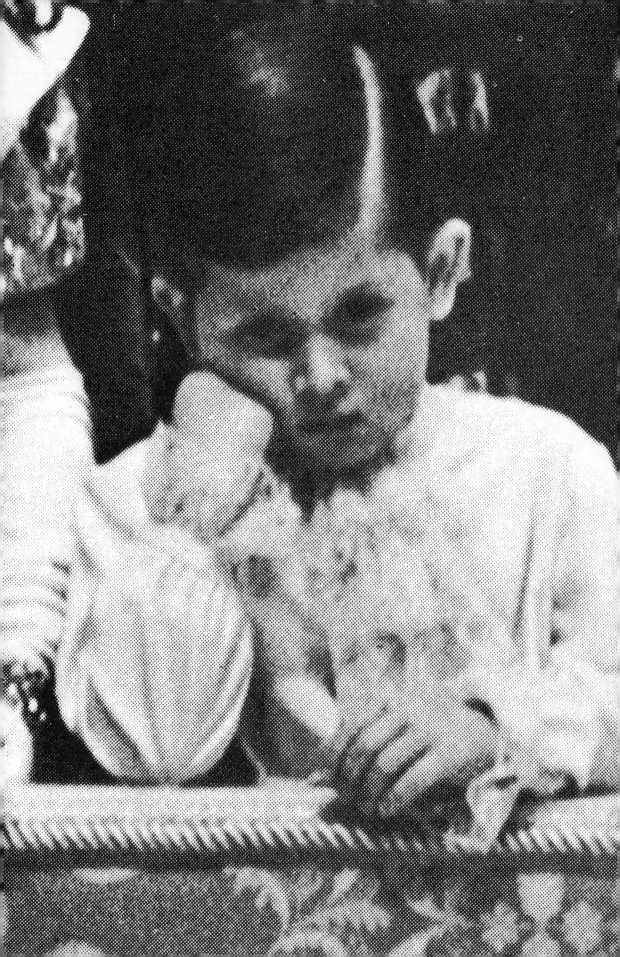

The Future King.

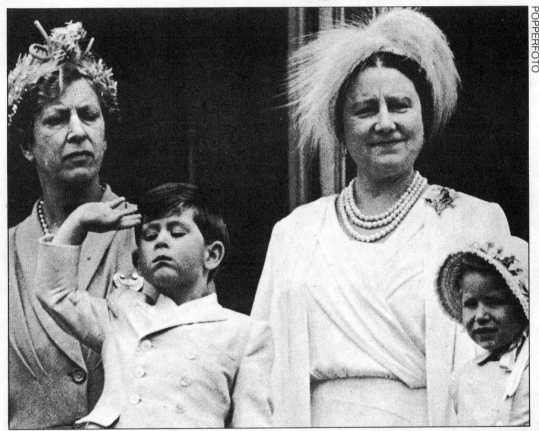

POPPERFOTO

I think it's something that dawns on you with the most ghastly, inexorable sense. I didn't suddenly wake up in my pram one day and say, "Yippee," you know.

First, I thought of being the proverbial engine driver. Then I wanted to grow up to be a sailor, as I had been on the yacht for the first time, and, of course, a soldier, because I had been watching the Changing of the Guard. When I started shooting, I thought how marvellous it would be to be a big-game hunter. I went from one thing to the other until I realised I was rather stuck.

I think it dawns on you slowly, that people are interested in you ... and slowly you get the idea that you have a certain duty and responsibility. I think it's better that way, rather than someone suddenly telling you, "You must do this," or, "You must do that," because you are who you are. I think it's one of those things you grow up in.

I might not be king for forty years, so I don't know what my role will be.

My great problem is that I don't really know what my role in life is. At the

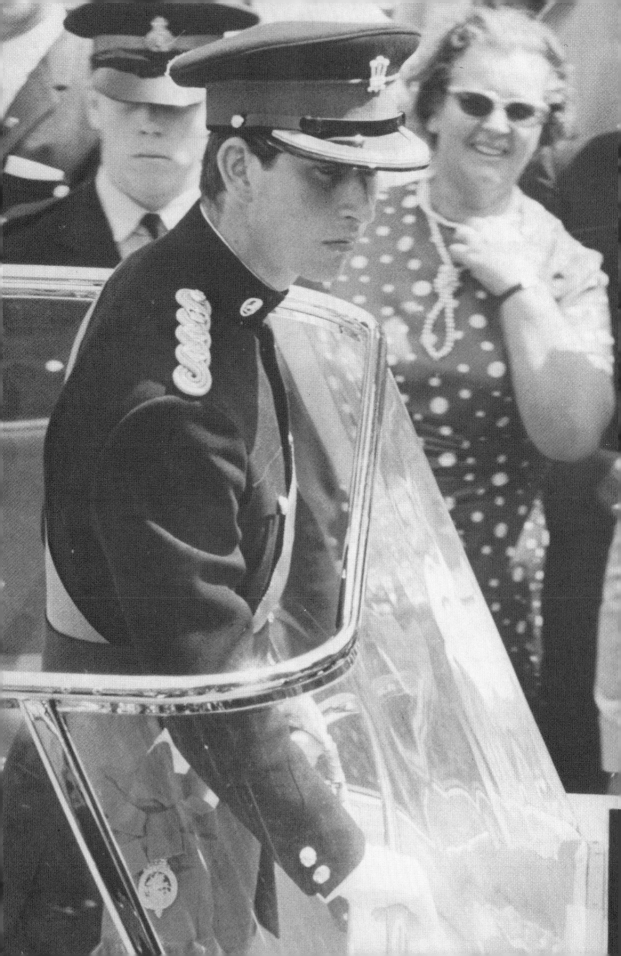

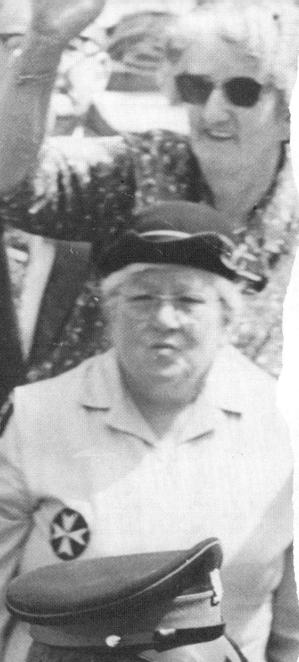

moment, I don't have one, but somehow I must find one for myself.

It's a fascinating job and I'm looking forward to the future.

I believe it best to confine myself to three basic aims at the start: to show concern for people, to display an interest in them as individuals, and to encourage them in a whole host of ways.

I've been trained to do it and I feel part of the job. I have this feeling of duty towards England, towards the United Kingdom

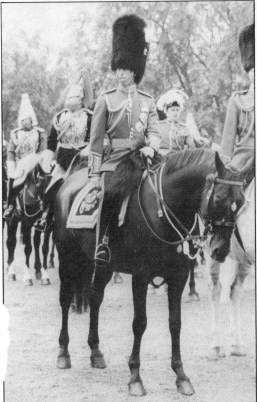

and towards the Commonwealth. I feel there's a great deal I can do if I'm given the chance to do it.

"I serve" is a marvellous motto to have, and I think that it's the basis of one's job.

If you have a sense of duty, and I like to think I have, then service is something that you give to people, particularly if they want you – but sometimes if they don't.

If you feel that you can do something… then you can be of service.

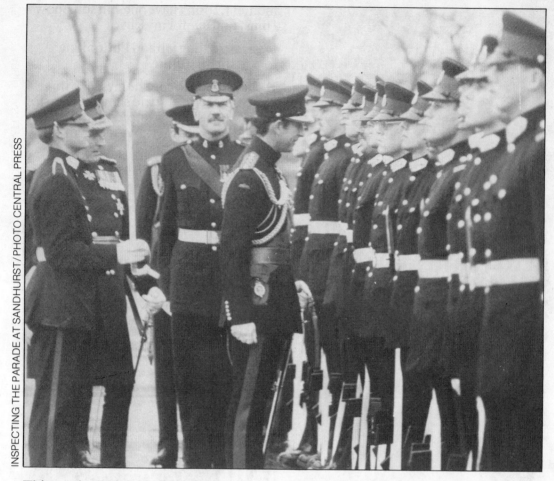

INSPECTING THE PARADE AT SANDHURST/PHOTO CENTRAL PRESS

This particular job is what I make it; you'll have to see what I do with it.

I think understanding on both sides is very important. I spend my life trying to understand others' problems. It's not easy, but I believe that it is most essential that one should have concern for people, help them get things off their chests.

I'm not much conscious of being a monarch-to-be. I'm much more conscious of being a Prince of Wales-as-is.

Yes, I suppose I *am* conscious of being different. You don't know – you can't know, can you? – how much different. After all, you only know what it is to be you, though you can study other people and deduce things about how *they* feel, to an extent.

But I've been brought up the way I have, and I've had the background I've had, and not many other people have had

that. So it does make one different, and make one feel different.

The most important thing for me is to have concern for people, to show it and provide some form of leadership.

I do worry about the future, but if one can preserve one's sense of humour, ability to adapt and, perhaps, help to calm things down and to provide a steadying influence, all will be well.

I think one has to be much more "with it" than of old, and much better informed.

I like to think I could be an ambassador not only for Wales, but also for the United Kingdom as a whole, and for one Commonwealth country to another.

I'm planning to find out all I can about British life, including the government, the civil service, agriculture, the unions and everything.

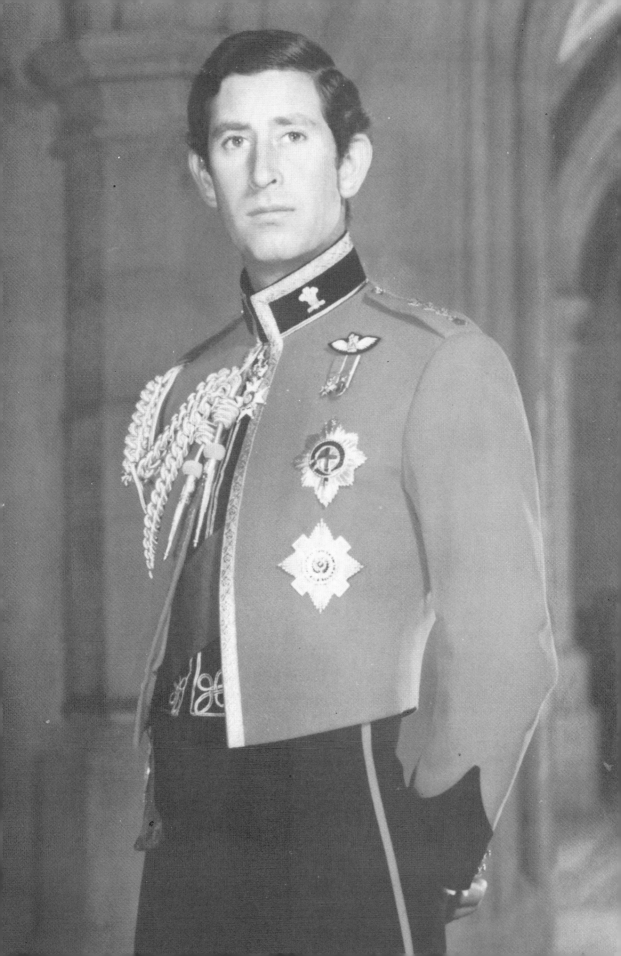

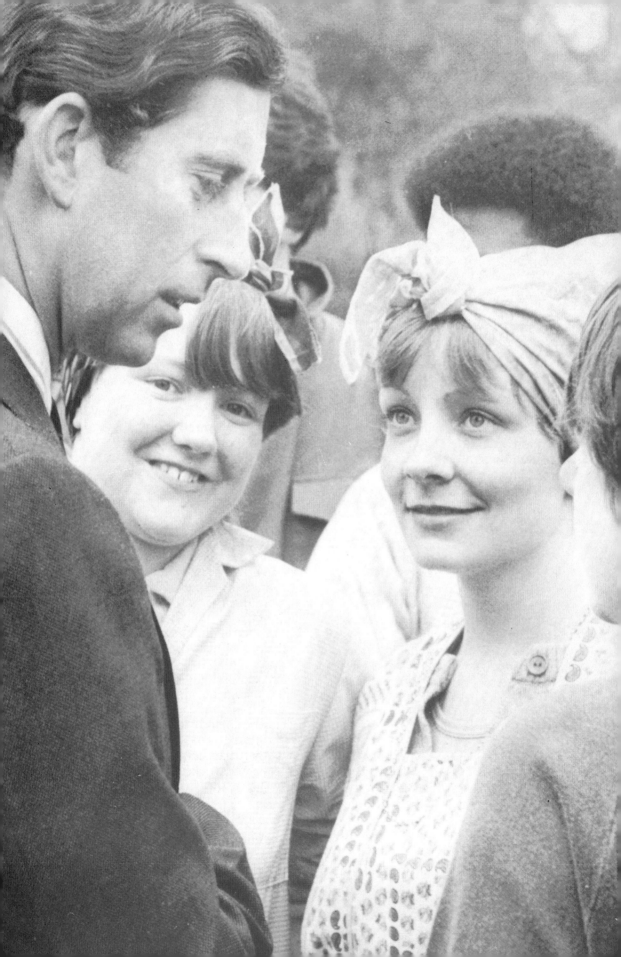

Britain & The British.

I've been all over the world and I always feel how marvellous it is to come back to Britain. You can read the papers when you're abroad and you think everything is coming to an end. But you discover that things are going on the same as always, and you feel happy to be back.

These things that are so important we take for granted ... our traditions and our institutions. This long tradition of basic freedom, which, in so many cases, doesn't exist in other countries.

We need to be reminded of these very important essential freedoms, which, more than any others, make Britain what it is to us and what it is to other people. All over the world, people look to Britain for an example and a lead in so many different ways.

The country's morale can be seriously harmed by what the media choose, or don't choose to emphasise.

The British are past masters at self-denigration. Practised reasonably, that's an attractive trait. But sometimes we go too far and are only reminded of the few things that we don't do well, like the strikes that occur in a small proportion of our industries, or the unpleasant things that foreigners say about us rather than the infinitely more frequent complimentary remarks which they make.

I remember only too well, somebody telling me that, regrettably, it doesn't make news that fifty jumbo jets landed safely at Heathrow Airport yesterday; but it does make news if one doesn't. I still believe, however, in the necessity of reminding people – metaphorically – that vast numbers of jumbo jets do land safely.

Britain has indulged in far more self-depreciation than is good for her. There are millions of people who work incredibly hard and achieve magnificent things without any recognition whatsoever.

The British react so marvellously to hard times. I love this country and want to see Britain great again.

I think the distinguishing characteristic of British people is their ability to laugh at themselves, to anticipate events. The British are inclined to accept the inevitable and to adapt themselves to changing circumstances.

Industry.

Britain is a modern, up-to-date society which is still in the forefront of technological and industrial advance – from nuclear power to Concorde.

In the past few years, it would be true to say Britain has had an unfortunate image overseas, certainly as far as her industrial relations are concerned. We are constantly told that we are going to the dogs and are finished as a nation, by various American television commentators.

In actual fact, things are not nearly so bad as they are made out to be. In a survey conducted in industrial countries by the International Labour Office, it was shown that the number of days lost per thousand workers in Britain was lower than in the United States.

I am sure there are some parts of British industry which are good at dealing with innovation, but there are an awful lot of good ideas simply not being adopted.

There are two possible reasons for this: either a new idea seems too risky, or a

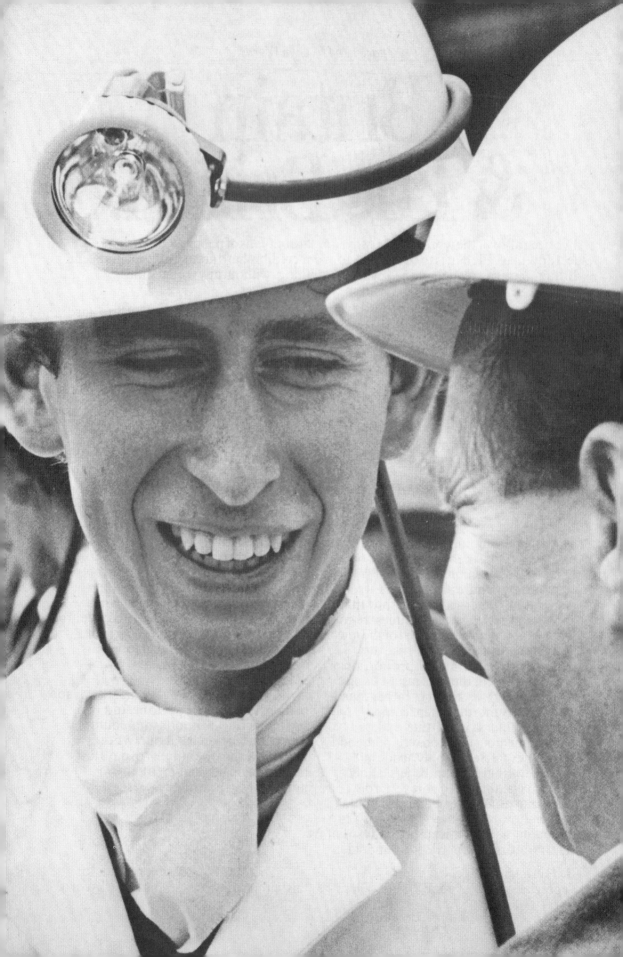

firm has its own ideas department which will jealously poo-poo anyone else's inspiration.

One of the great problems in Britain is to produce a marketable product from an invention. It seems people in Japan, France and America are much better at that than we are.

Charles speaks out:

I have not the slightest hesitation in making the observation that much of British manufacturing does not seem to understand the importance of the human factor.

I discovered during my recent visits that the problem of communication between management and the shop floor frequently stems from a failure of communications within management.

When front line managers are accused of poor communications, the truth is often that they cannot communicate because they don't know much themselves.

There is a sense in which the British managements remain inclined to play their cards very close to their chest in respect of company performance and plans.

This is not calculated to gain trust and co-operation from the work-force, which is essential if they are to co-operate with the introduction of change. People are not impossible to deal with.

Good British factories are very good, by any standards. The trouble is that there are not enough good ones. Why? Because the communication structure is inadequate.

A shop-stewards' convenor told of a manager who breezed in in the morning with a pipe firmly in the teeth, never bothered to acknowledge anyone and gave instructions to everyone. When he had a problem they all told him to get stuffed – probably through their shop floor supervisor.

British management might have something to learn from America. Their "single status" system, which is now beginning to be adopted by certain British companies, has a great deal to recommend it. Basically, it means that the conditions of employment are the same whatever your position.

It also means eating in the same canteen.

Engineering:

Greater liaison and co-operation is necessary between industry and education in order to drag large parts of British manufacturing industry into the competitive 1980's.

British schools give high status to abstract learning and, as a result, practical experts like engineers have suffered a low status in Britain compared to overseas.

Engineers are too often seen as people who wear overalls, wield spanners and do dirty, undignified jobs.

What is badly needed, is action rather than sweet words. The various engineering organisations should stop arguing about who should be entitled to initiate any changes.

What is at stake, I believe, is the future success and potential prosperity of this country. If this arguing continues, there will be a distinct danger of becoming hopelessly bogged down and the best chance we have had for a long time...will be irrevocably lost.

The reason for my interest and concern is based on a simple observation: if we are going to regenerate industry in this country, to compete anywhere near successfully with our major competitors, and to create sufficient wealth to pay for such expensive luxuries as universities and all the other facilities we take for granted in modern society, then we have no alternative but to improve the status of the engineer and encourage those whose skills are essential to the manufacturing potential of the United Kingdom.

Attitudes in schools are crucial and the new degree course in electronic and electrical engineering at Bath was a bold initiative.

But many other universities were slow in introducing more practical and relevant subjects in response to the demand of a modern, technological society. There is definitely what can be described only as a "stick-in-the-mud" attitude in this sphere on the part of many universities.

I pray this will soon change to a positive realisation that adaptation to new and challenging circumstances *must* take place if we are to remain a major trading nation. Industry should not leave education to the academics and should make more practical training places available to graduates.

Engineers' skills are just as valuable as those of other professions, such as doctors and lawyers, but they have still not been recognised as such.

Our aim, therefore, should be to give potential engineers the chance they deserve and the moral encouragement they need so badly.

Reluctance and in-built conservatism would merely lead to a Pyrrhic victory for engineering. Nothing would be done and in the late twentieth century we'd merely find ourselves as one of the minor industrial states with no voice in international affairs, treated with pity, and, no doubt, with ridicule from time to time.

When asked to open a factory "very informally":
You mean you want me to drive a fork-lift truck through the wall?

On being addressed as "Charlie" by Yorkshire miners' leader, Joe Gormley:
I'm delighted to be called Charlie. It's better than the woman who jumped out of a crowd the other day and said, "Look, there's Action Man." It's better than in America, where they called you "prince." You do get fed up with being referred to like an RAF police dog.

Things are tending to change too quickly. People haven't had time to catch up

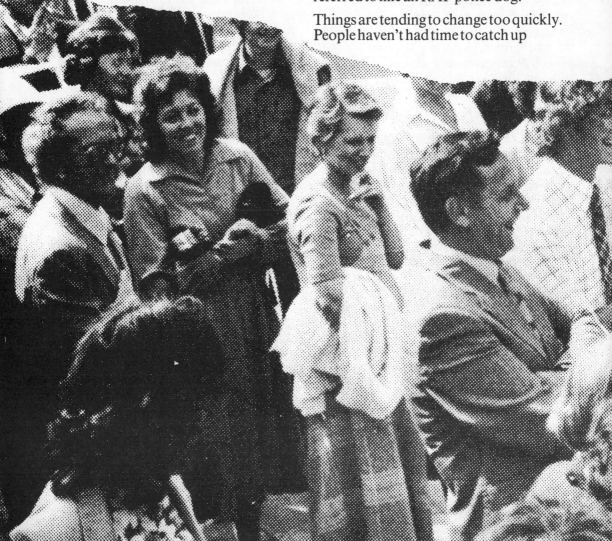

psychologically. This poses problems of all sorts: people don't really know where they stand; they don't know what's going to happen next and they can't plan for the future; they can't look ahead. Rapid change is something I find difficult to keep up with.

I believe strongly that one should adapt to changes, particularly in my position. You can't afford to get left miles behind.

Likewise, you don't want to be too far ahead. I think you always want to be just a little bit behind, but adapting gently and slowly, in some cases, taking the initiative and doing something before it's forced on you.

If you are taking it in the strictly economic sense, our competitors have managed to change much quicker than we have.

Mainly, it's because we were one of the few nations at the end of the last war that didn't actually lose out, so to speak. I come to the conclusion, looking around, that those who came off worst in the war had to change quickest.

It's an ugly fact to face sometimes, that economics, whether you like it or not, are here to stay. If you live in this particular world, you have to exist by trading and competing.

If you want, we can all drop out and live on little plots of land. Everybody may be much happier, but they're jolly well not going to have the things that we have now and that we take for granted – television, washing machines, cars and all these things. How the hell do they think we have all these, if it's not through our ability to produce the wealth to pay for them?

PHOTO METAL CONSTRUCTION

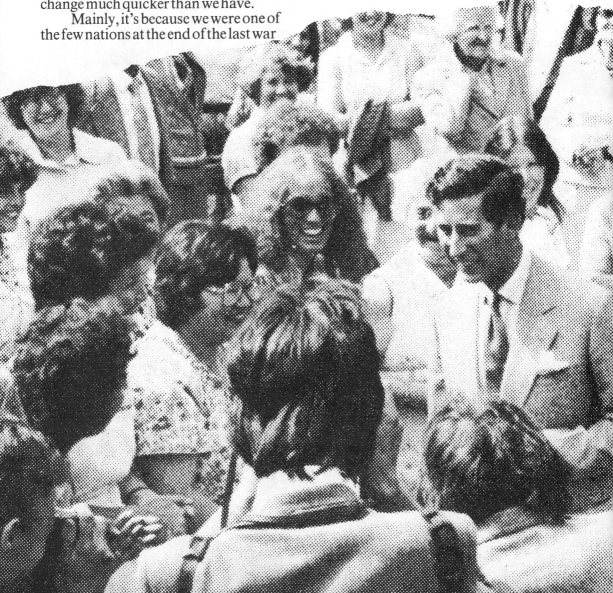

Young People.

I believe strongly that many more young people should be given the opportunity to find excitement and adventure through voluntary service and by organising themselves after initial help and training.

There are certainly plenty of things that young people could do, which involve an adventurous challenge and the responsibility of adulthood at a time when it's flattering and important to be considered as an adult.

    The important thing is that the young people should run their own show. They don't want to do things which are planned and supervised by adults.

I often feel that in urban areas there's a distinct lack of facilities for younger people. I feel sometimes that the kind of attitude you see – particularly, for instance, at football matches – is really that they're trying to get rid of pent-up energy and enthusiasm. To my mind, it is misdirected.

    I feel that they could be given opportunities – not just going to a football match, but other things – where they can get rid of their energy.

    It's a problem that's always been with us, but more noticeably since the end of National Service.

Now, there's a limit as to how much of the adventure young people want can be combined with useful work.

    But I'm sure you'll wave goodbye to any sense of adventure if you ask them to do only things that are suggested, laid on and directed by grown-ups. Especially by grown-ups who come from what they regard as "the Establishment" – the leaders of organisations which have been with us for many years – and are regarded, rightly or wrongly, by these young people as being hampered by class, religion or even a political outlook and background to which the young people don't subscribe.

    It's not so much that they oppose these older people; they just feel they are remote, irrelevant.

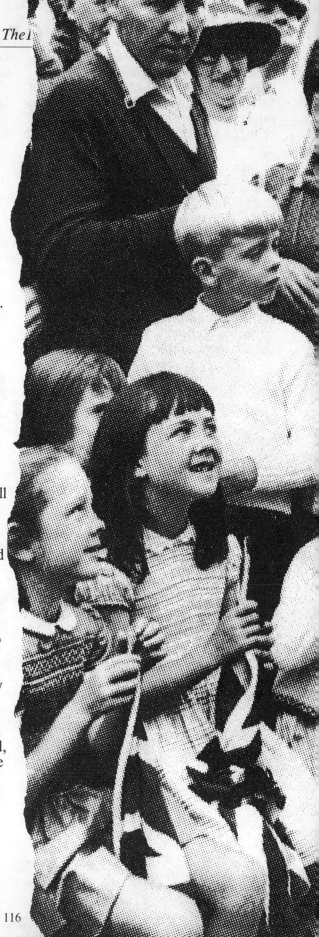

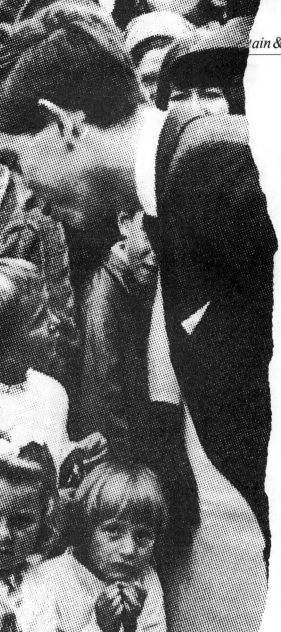

PHOTO THE SUN

Youth: it's an awful word, really. Let's say "young people."

I'm now old enough, and I've seen enough, to worry about the alienation of young people from adult society. It's mainly in London and the big cities: I don't think it's so tough in the country.

What's wrong is that so many young people feel they don't belong, because they don't have a sense of service, of contributing. In the cities, the young coloured people feel this even more strongly.

The Queen's Silver Jubilee Appeal.

The central idea is this: there'd be a trust holding the funds.

Young people – including existing organisations – would come to the trust and say, "We want to do this. Will you give us the money?" The trust could then examine proposals; if they thought they'd work, they'd say, "Right, there's the money, and any help we can give. Get on with it."

Before we set up the trust – before it accepts the money which I believe is now available – we must be sure that the method will work and that enough young people will come forward to take advantage of it.

So, at the moment, there are pilot schemes being planned – one in Wales, one in Cornwall, one in London.

If they succeed, you'll hear more about the idea soon – and the trust will come into being, and work along those general lines.

Finance has to be supplied. There's got to be a certain amount of initial adult activity if the young people's projects are going to be launched. But as soon as they have got their own thing going, leave them alone.

I feel there's an alternative to bashing each other up at football matches, or whatever it is. It's just a question of getting them involved in more exciting things.

I happen to feel that you can involve more of the difficult type of person who one doesn't normally get to through the

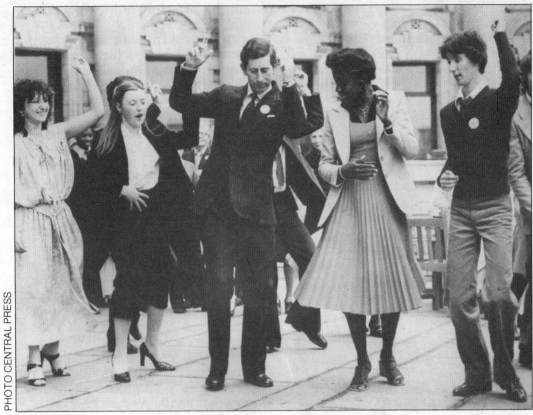

medium of existing youth organisations. A lot of them are looking for kicks in some way or another and the kicks can be directed in a useful way.

There are lots of things chaps with motorcycles can do.

Let's help young blacks. Let's help the young help the old. All that goes without saying, but do you think there's anything we can do to help in Northern Ireland?

Immigration.

With supreme disregard for the dictates of caution and diplomacy, I urged that a great deal of good could be achieved by well-made films, primarily to explain to people living in this country the reasons for our behaviour, and to show the similarities that exist – even in the apparent differences between ourselves and other races.

My belief rested on the feeling that, if only more people could have the advantages of information and knowledge about other people's social behaviour, customs, religion and so forth, then perhaps some of the prejudice against immigrant groups in this country might be slowly reduced.

The more people understood about the background of our immigrants, the less apprehensive they would be about them. To get on neighbourly terms with people of other races and countries, you've got to get more familiar with them – know how they live, how they eat, how they work, what makes them laugh, their history.

I'm particularly fortunate in having seen different people in their own environments – many of which I have admired and found fascinating. It's easier, therefore, for me not to be prejudiced.

But it's difficult not to be prejudiced if they come and live in your street, and possibly the value of your property falls because of the new people arriving, and if you believe all the bad things you're told about them, because you don't know any better.

You can't remove people's apprehensions in one night, but you can make a start by making them more knowledgeable. If the Anthropological Society can help us to do that, I'm going to help it.

We hope to stimulate interest and knowledge and tolerance through new TV programmes – this is a field in which TV can be of immense assistance. Given that, as I say, you can't change attitudes or facts overnight, or in a year, you *can* speed up the rate at which people's minds change.

If you want examples of what I'd like to do in general, one thing is helping people and organisations to give us all more information about the problems we face as individual citizens.

Whatever cause I associate with, I want to *participate*.

Some organisations would be quite happy to have me as, say, patron, and just put my name on the literature. But I want to *do* something for it, with it, and through it.

I don't want to be a figure-head. I want to help get things done.

Wales.

In Wales, there isn't so much of a middle class as there is in England. The extraordinary thing about Welshmen is that they have this radical tradition – they are radically traditional and traditionally radical, and this is a curious paradox. They have an old tradition of support for the Labour Party, for instance, and yet, in the country regions, they are also very traditional in the more general sense of the word.

There's a certain amount of truth in saying that Wales has been neglected by a central government – it's on the fringes, and this has led to a certain depressed feeling and perhaps a slight inferiority complex, I'm not sure. At the same time, in Wales, as a result of their union with England, the upper strata of society moved off to England, and as it were relinquished their responsibilities towards the ordinary people.

As a result, the people of Wales have established their own folk culture, their own music, eisteddfods and folk dancing. Everything like that is unique to Wales, an essential part of the Welsh character.

England hasn't got anything like it.

Somebody was asking me the other day how England would like it if a Welshman was made Prince of England. Well, I don't think, in fact, English people would worry as much as the Welsh. It's not the same.

When I went to Llanelli not long ago, the mayor said, "Can you say 'Llanelli'?" I said; "Llanelli?," and he wiped the saliva out of his eye and said, "Well done."

I want to see as many people as possible in Wales show that they love their country as much as they say and sing they do.

The Commonwealth.

I don't think it would be a disaster if Britain withdrew from the Commonwealth; I'm sure it could survive without Britain. But I believe that the Queen, as head of the Commonwealth, plays an important part in keeping the whole thing together.

It's a wider family than it was and it is the Commonwealth and not the British Commonwealth. Too often, people are inclined to treat the concept of the Commonwealth with cynicism, or to reject it altogether as an anachronism and complete waste of everybody's time and effort.

Above all, I believe it is up to the young people of the Commonwealth to show that they believe that association has something to offer the modern world, because without their support, interest and encouragement, it will only be a matter of time before the whole thing fades away through lack of interest.

The whole question fascinates me. There's an enormous amount to be done there; the Commonwealth is one of those associations which require a great deal of effort and expertise to make it work satisfactorily and usefully in world terms.

I think there must be something unique about it, in that it has remained in being as long as it has. There must be some deep bond that's worth developing.

There must be something to be said for the Commonwealth, after all.

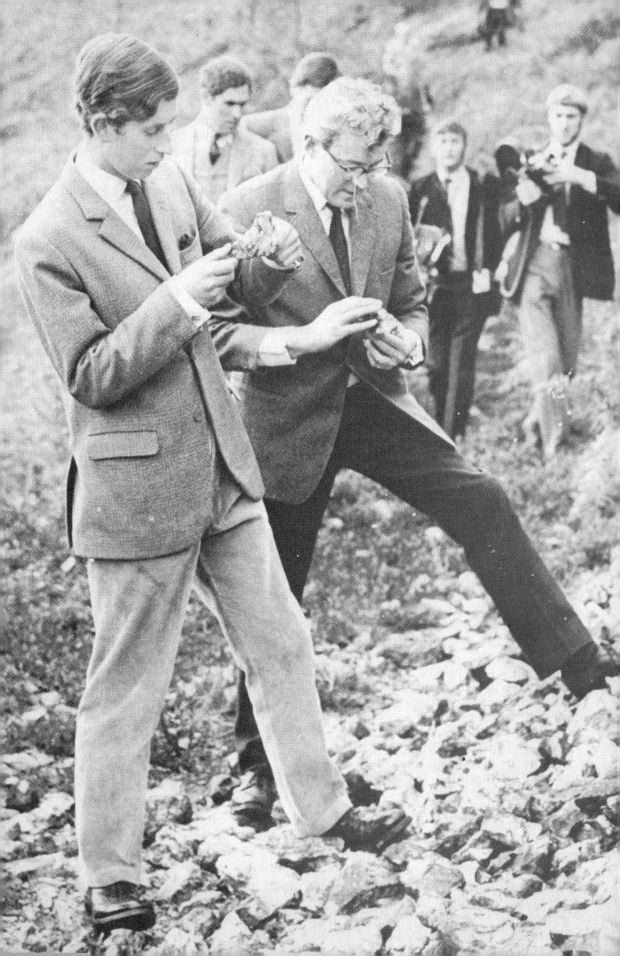

Ecology.

The future of our planet depends on the interest and involvement of the young in projects which improve the environment. Any work to improve the environment in the next few years would meet serious economic difficulties. We'll be faced with hard decisions about priorities.

It's not an impossible thing to achieve as long as it's realised that the countryside will not just stay here, serene and beautiful, unless countless individuals are determined it should do so.

We can achieve nothing without the immensely useful co-operation of the public and of the people who use the country most.

The aim is to create awareness that efforts in conservation and pollution control are designed for the long-term good of this country. To go on virtually destroying what we live in, until the final horror really strikes us, and then try to do something is

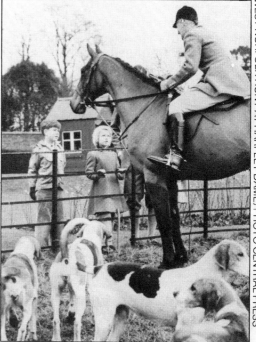

WEST NORFOLK HUNT AT HARPLEY DAME/PHOTO CENTRAL PRESS

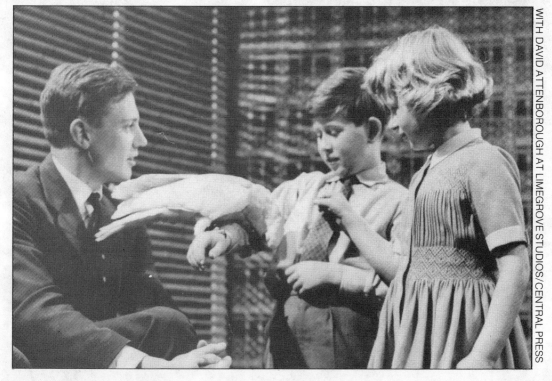

WITH DAVID ATTENBOROUGH AT LIMEGROVE STUDIOS/CENTRAL PRESS

surely an insult to human rational thinking.

Charles was very impressed with the Canadian north:

Our own particular civilisation, if you can call it that, loses a great deal in an attempt to control nature. We must always remember that we are basically animals – and not to destroy any more of nature than is absolutely necessary.

Hunting:

I deeply revel in nature. I really do enjoy animals as such. It's part of man's curious instinct over thousands of years to go hunting – perhaps there is something wrong with my breeding.

Because you kill animals doesn't mean that you don't appreciate them fully or want to conserve them.

I think that if people did not partake in country sports in this country, there

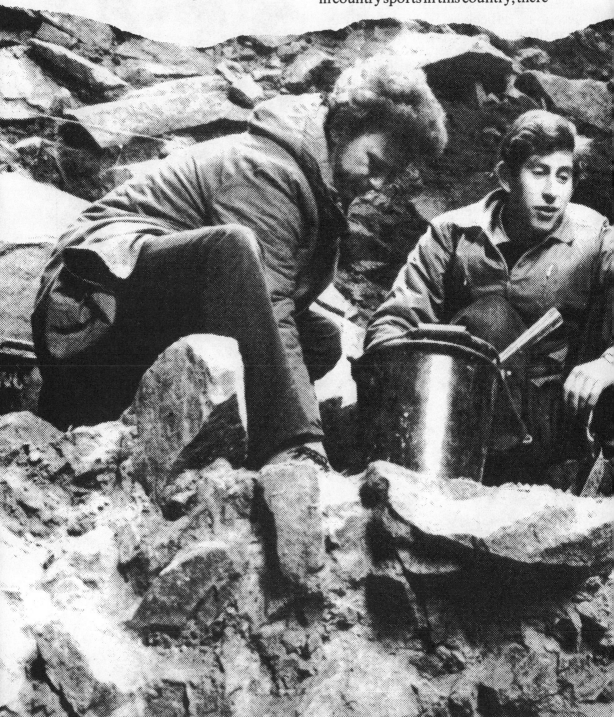

would not be many animals left. There would not be the countryside we have now. It would be a basically average desert because most farmers would plough up hedges for more productive land.

It's because so many people enjoy hunting and shooting that the country remains as it is.

Cars:

Society committed to a machine that requires tracks to be scoured across the increasingly precious countryside, can either shrug its shoulders and excuse unoriginal and unimaginative road-building, or press for designs which harmonise, as far as possible, with the natural features of the countryside.

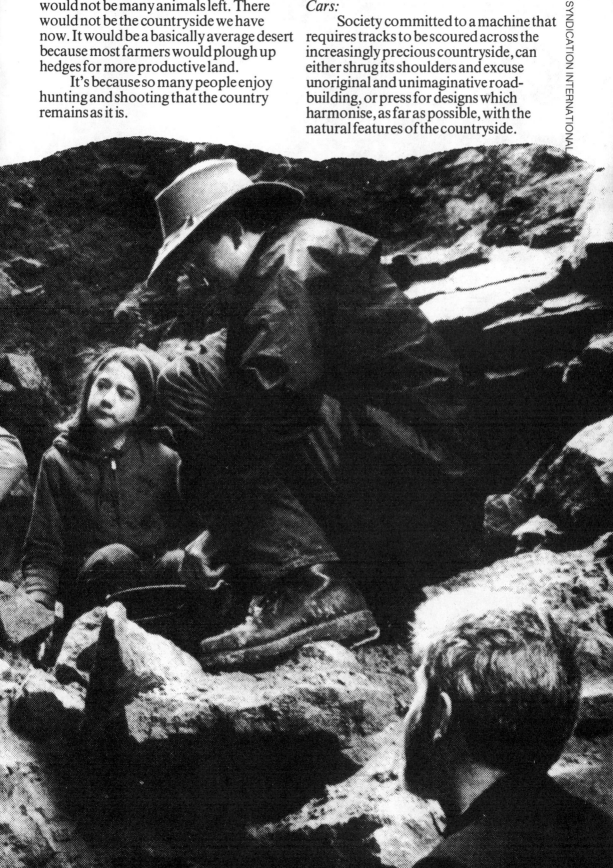

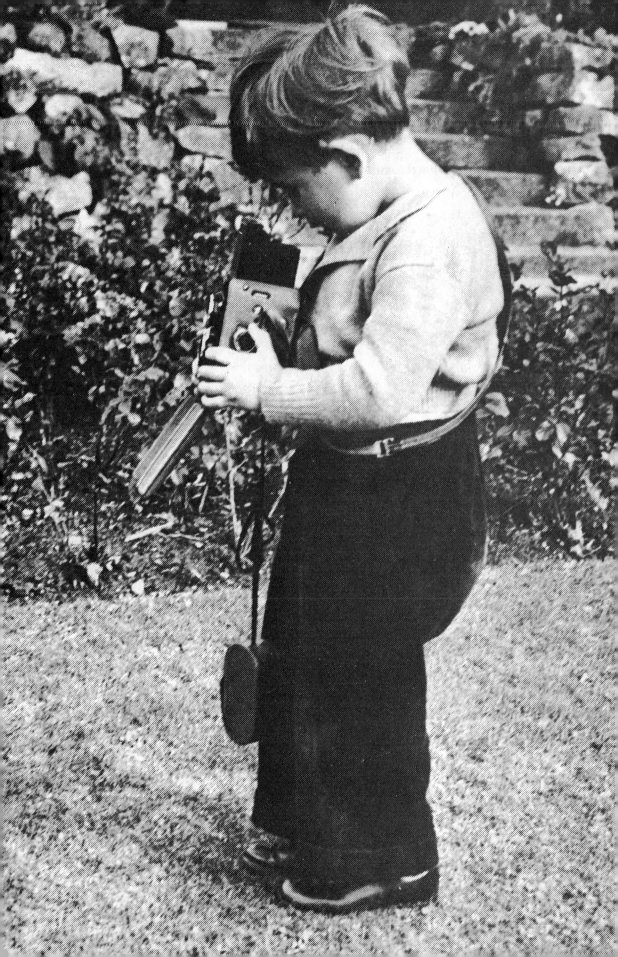

The Press.

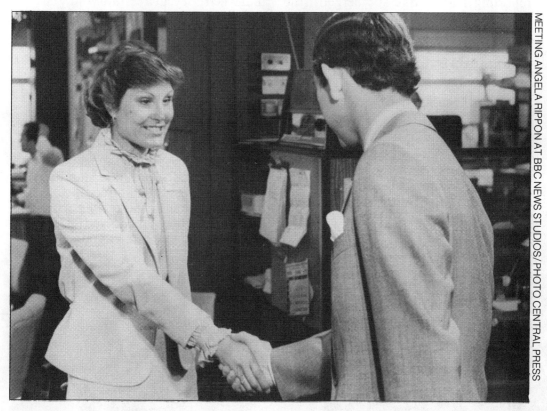

Haven't you got enough pictures now?

However much one might inveigh against the Press – personally and collectively – I came to the conclusion long ago that there is always a price to be paid for freedom. A free Press is as much a part and a guarantor of our civilisation and liberty as any other factor.

There is, therefore, no question about the importance of a free Press in the world of the mid-Seventies. The right to report and criticise freely was hard won.

Charles composed this Ode to the Press while in Canada:

Impossible, unapproachable, God only
    knows,
The light's always dreadful and he won't
    damn-well pose,
Most maddening, most curious, he simply
    can't fail,

It's always the same with the old Prince
    of Wales.

Insistent, persistent, the Press never end,
One day they will drive me right round
    the bend,
Recording, rephrasing, every word
    that I say,
It's got to be news at the end of the day.

Disgraceful, most dangerous to share
    the same plane,
Denies me the chance to scratch and
    complain,
Oh where, may I ask, is the Monarchy
    going,
When Princes and pressmen are on
    the same Boeing?

The programme's so formal and highly
    arranged,
But haven't you heard that it's all been
    changed,

Friday is Sunday and that is quite plain,
So no one, please no one, is allowed
to complain.

Honesty and integrity are vital factors (in
reporting) and often get submerged in the
general rush for sensationalism. The
media has a large responsibility for the
news it presents. The important thing is
for truth to be actually portrayed.

The less people know about what is really
going on, the easier it is to wield power and
authority.

While many journalists approach their
job with a strong sense of responsibility,
the temptations to indulge in cynicism,
sarcasm or sensationalism must be
enormous. People believe what they read

in the papers. Even I find myself soaking
up what the pages of print tell me.

I have read so many reports recently
telling everyone who I am about to marry,
that when last year a certain young lady
was staying at Sandringham, a crowd of
about ten thousand appeared when we
went to church.

Such was the obvious conviction
that what they read was true I almost
felt I had better espouse myself at once so
as not to disappoint too many people.
As you can see, I thought better of it.

From my sister's point of view, the
behaviour of the photographers is very
hard to take, and I can understand why.
If you're doing something competitive in
public, especially in the top international
class, you are inevitably keyed up. To have
a lot of people with cameras pursuing you,

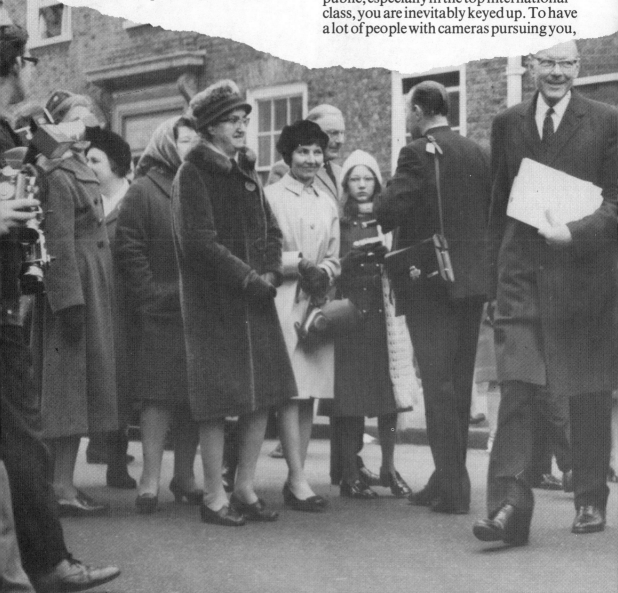

and possibly frightening the horse, is annoying, to say the least.

It is easy to become irritable and to feel that it is only when things go wrong – when you are upside down or halfway up a tree – that photographs appear in the paper or on TV.

When I was younger, I sometimes used to get cross. Then, as I got older, I tried to think it out. I knew I mustn't go on being cross or shouting at people – it wasn't becoming in one so young.

So I tried to understand the other person's position and put myself in his shoes. Part of that means recognising the demands a newspaper makes of all the people who work on it, even if they own it.

Anyway, it's when nobody wants to write about you or take a photograph of you that you ought to worry in my sort of job.

Then there would be no point in being around – and I couldn't stand being around if there didn't seem to be any point to it.

Those foreign papers will report anything. One of them said I was having an affair with someone or other, the other day.

They are incredibly disreputable, but everybody reads them. They know it's nonsense but they love reading them.

Sometimes, particularly trivial stories about me appear. I suppose I must accept that what happens to me can be newsworthy, regardless of the context.

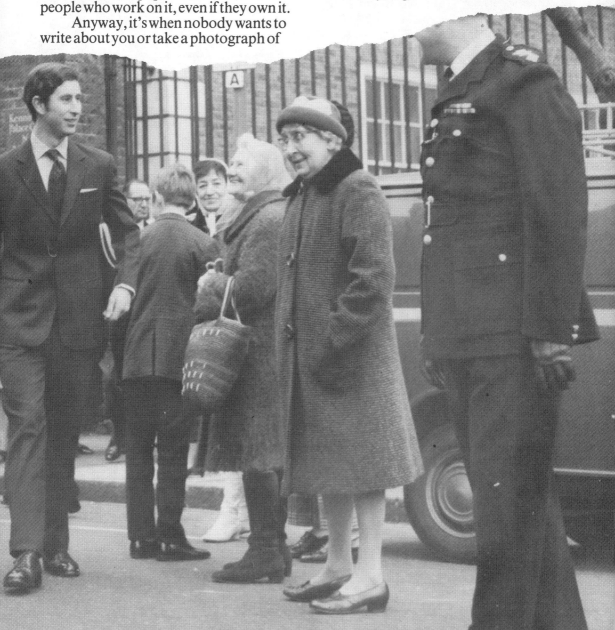

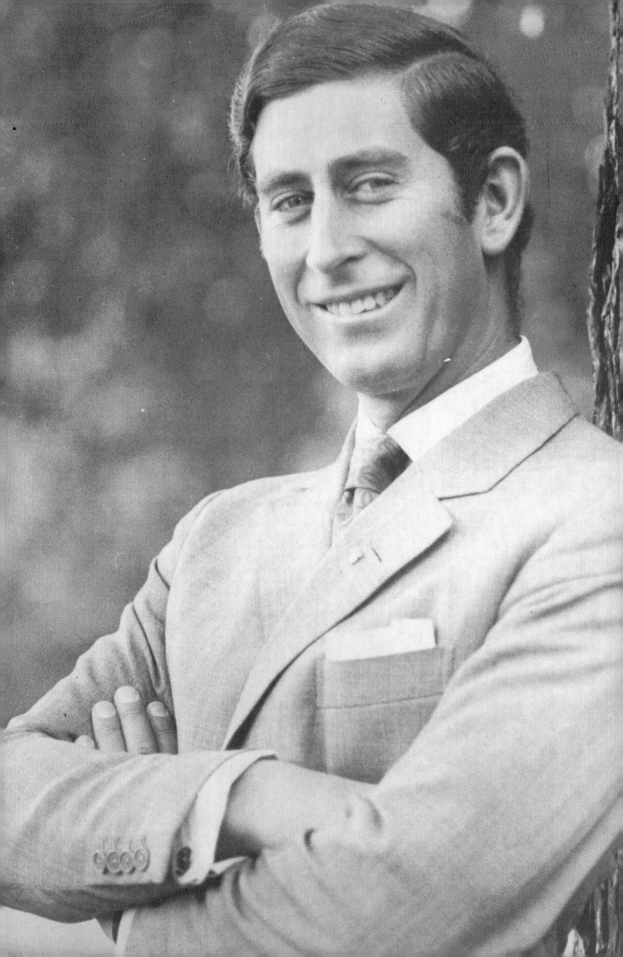